Doing Research

Martha E. Farrar Highfield

Doing Research

A Practical Guide for Health
Professionals

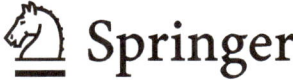 Springer

Martha E. Farrar Highfield
Nursing
California State University
Northridge, CA, USA

Nursing
Providence Holy Cross Medical Center
Mission Hills, CA, USA

ISBN 978-3-031-79043-0   ISBN 978-3-031-79044-7   (eBook)
https://doi.org/10.1007/978-3-031-79044-7

This Springer imprint is published by the registered company Springer Nature Switzerland AG
The registered company address is: Gewerbestrasse 11, 6330 Cham, Switzerland

If disposing of this product, please recycle the paper.

To my research mentees, who teach me how to make the difficult simple.

Preface

Do you have a burning clinical research question, but little or no research experience? If so, and you need a step-by-step summary of how to do research, then this book is for you. It explains what research is and isn't, where to begin and end, and the meaning of key terms. A project planning worksheet is included.

The purpose of this book is to empower curious clinicians who want data-based answers. To get the most from *Doing Research*, first review its table of contents, figures, and boxes. Then as you read through the book, complete the Protocol Worksheet. Focus on what *you* need to know.

Doing Research is a user-friendly guide, not a comprehensive text. Chapter 1 gives a dozen tips to get started, Chap. 2 defines research, and Chaps. 3, 4, 5, 6, 7, 8 and 9 focus on planning. The remaining Chaps. 10, 11 and 12 guide you through challenges of conducting a study, getting answers from the data, and sharing with others what you learned. Italicized key terms are defined in the glossary, and a bibliography lists additional resources.

I gratefully acknowledge my "book village." Among them are statistician Ross Bindler PharmD, residency director Henry Farrar III MD, and novice researchers Deepti Bhatnagar RN, MSN, MBA and Susan Egami MSN RNC-NIC IBCLC, each of whom reviewed the manuscript in part or whole. I am thankful, too, for Carolyn L. Cason PhD RN FAAN who decades ago started me down a research path that I never imagined and for colleagues Mara Raggi MSN NE-BC RNC-NIC and Ann DeChairo-Marino PhD RN NEA-BC who opened new doors to me in clinical research. Finally, I am grateful for the support of my husband Ron and sons Nathanael and Matthew and for the legacy of my late parents Henry Farrar Jr MD and Grace Johnson Farrar RN who taught me in word and deed never to back down from a worthwhile challenge.

Northridge & Mission Hills, CA, USA   Martha E. Farrar Highfield

Contents

About the Author

Martha E. Farrar Highfield PhD RN is Professor Emeritus of Nursing at California State University/Northridge (CSUN) and advisor for nurse research fellows at Providence Holy Cross Medical Center in Mission Hills, California. Her experience encompasses over four decades of research, teaching, administrative, and clinical experience in both public and private settings. She has presented locally, nationally, and internationally, and authored numerous peer-reviewed articles, two professional book chapters, and one historical research book. In 2003 she received the Outstanding Nursing Alumnus Award from Harding University's Carr College of Nursing, and in 2012 received the Extraordinary Faculty Service Award from CSUN. Dr. Highfield (or "Dr H" to her students) holds membership in the American Association for History of Nursing and Sigma Theta Tau International Nursing Honor Society. Online profiles are on LinkedIn and ResearchGate, and she authors a blog for clinical staff: Discovering Your Inner Scientist (https://discoveringyourinnerscientist.com/). Her email is martha.highfield@csun.edu.

A Dozen Tips to Start

1

As you begin your research journey, remember that it's more like a marathon than a sprint. Here are 12 tips to get started.

1. **Don't go it alone.** Combine your experiential knowledge with the technical expertise of a research mentor. If you are clinical staff, find out if your planned research site has an established mentoring pathway. If you are a student, faculty will provide academic mentoring.
2. **Don't undervalue your existing knowledge.** Direct care clinicians see problems firsthand that expert researchers may miss, and vice versa.
3. **Don't overvalue your existing knowledge.** Research is about discovering what we don't know—it's not about proving opinions. Ask for guidance, and listen. Constructive criticism means that the person invested time in your success.
4. **Pick a topic you love.** This will keep you energized during tedious moments. When (not if) you hit "researcher's block," do something to rekindle your interest, like talking to an encouraging peer or taking a walk. See also #5.
5. **Take "baby steps."** Do at least one thing toward project completion each day, no matter how tiny. One investigator joked about adding a period one day, and deleting it the next.
6. **Be patient.** A research project takes months to years. A rare few can be done within weeks.

© The Author(s), under exclusive license to Springer Nature Switzerland AG 2025
M. E. F. Highfield, *Doing Research*,
https://doi.org/10.1007/978-3-031-79044-7_1

7. **Don't procrastinate.** Reject distractions like email, social media, or cleaning your desk. Write down your ideas; don't just talk about them. Set a timer, and work for at least 10 minutes. As Nike says, "Just do it."

8. **Take a class.** Enroll in research-related classes offered by your institution, or check out free material online. You'll either learn a lot or get a confidence boost when you find out how much you already know.

9. **Write your protocol using your research-site or university IRB template.** A *protocol* is the written step-by-step plan for conducting your study. The *IRB* (*institutional review board*) is an ethics committee who must legally approve your protocol before the study begins. Using an IRB template speeds approval. Consult your mentor if you need to choose between full or minimal risk templates or between facility IRBs.

10. **Remember: No study is perfect.** You will not conduct a perfect study. No one ever has. Nonetheless, you should meticulously plan protocol details in terms of the who, what, when, where, and how of your study. Then, after study completion be ruthlessly honest in reporting your project's limitations and strengths, so that your findings can be well-used.

11. **Planning a study never moves in a straight line.** Don't be surprised if you find yourself moving back and forth between steps. As you learn, don't hesitate to improve your protocol.

12. **If this is your first research project, consider a descriptive study.** Descriptive studies are simpler; they usually involve one-time data collection to describe an existing situation. Intervention studies are more complicated, requiring you to collect data often from two or more groups, try out an intervention, and collect data again. That said, if you love your intervention topic, stick with it!

  Next step: Some basics

What Research Is (& Is Not)

2

Research yields knowledge that facilitates giving the right care in the right way at the right time in the right place to the right person. Of course not every clinician needs to conduct research, but caregivers often confront issues that need data-based solutions. Merely asking colleagues how they resolve a clinical issue limits you to what those particular individuals know—or think they know. And besides, research can be fun!

2.1 What Is Research?

Simply put, *research* is a systematic way to ask and answer questions by finding patterns in new or existing data. Its purpose is to discover *generalizable* knowledge. A specific type, *human subjects research*, engages with identifiable, living individuals or their private information.

2.1.1 Research Process

Figure 2.1 illustrates the research process, including stating the problem, planning, gaining IRB approval, conducting the study, and disseminating results. Planning especially is a back-and-forth process.

© The Author(s), under exclusive license to Springer Nature Switzerland AG 2025   3
M. E. F. Highfield, *Doing Research*,
https://doi.org/10.1007/978-3-031-79044-7_2

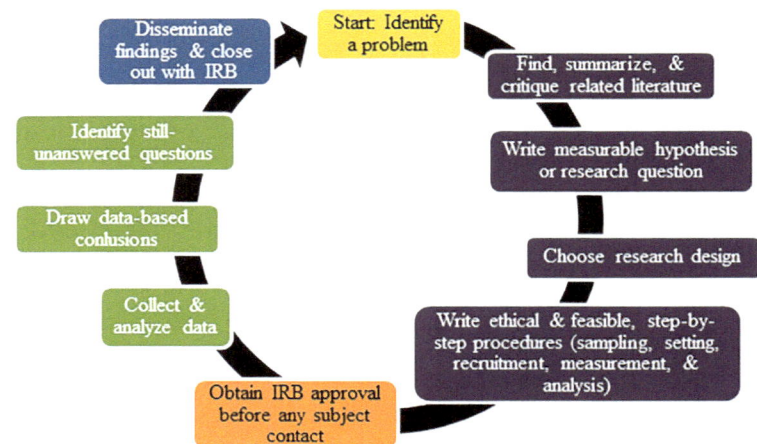

Fig. 2.1   Research process

Also, the final step of sharing results (dissemination) is as important as any other. Every completed study leads to new questions, and the Fig. 2.1 cycle is repeated.

Two complementary types of research follow the Fig. 2.1 cycle: Basic research and applied research. Your project is one or the other. First, curiosity-driven basic researchers investigate something for its own sake, and second, applied researchers use that basic information to test practical solutions. Together basic and applied research findings build clinical knowledge. An example is when basic research describes underserved children's nutritional status, and then applied research tests the effectiveness of a particular dietary intervention for them.

Both basic and applied researchers start the Fig. 2.1 process by identifying an issue that is worth the time and effort to study. After that, they read topic-related literature, articulate a yet-to-be-answered hypothesis or question (H/Q), and design a study that guides data gathering and analysis to answer that H/Q.

Hypotheses and questions are different. A *hypothesis* is a theory-derived, research-informed prediction about the relationship between two or more variables—here called X and Y. A hypothesis might be "[X treatment] will improve [Y outcome]." In contrast when researchers do not have enough information to hypothesize, they ask *research questions*, such as "What are characteristics of [X]?" or "Are [X] and [Y] related?"

The *variables* in H/Qs are things that occur in different amounts or qualities. In other words, variables vary! Researchers measure those variations, analyze the measurements, and draw conclusions. Variables may be measured as binary options (e.g., cleft palate or no cleft palate), as numbers (e.g., weight in pounds), as categories (e.g., languages of English, Farsi, Tagalog), as stages of a process (e.g., grief), or as themes and meanings (e.g., the experience of parenting twins). Moreover, the same variable may be measured differently; for example, blood pressure can be measured by sphygmomanometer, arterial line, or patient self-report.

Data (singular *datum*) are the numerical or nonnumerical measurements of variables. Numerical measurements are called *quantitative data* and are analyzed statistically. Nonnumerical measurements are *qualitative data* and are analyzed through critical reflection; examples of qualitative data include transcribed interviews and historical photographs.

> **Alert!** When investigators measure the same variable differently, their research findings may conflict. This means more study is needed.

Researchers may collect data *prospectively* as new data or *retrospectively* as existing data. An example of existing data are laboratory results that were collected for clinical diagnoses not research. In prospective studies, researchers have more control over how and what data are gathered, and so prospective research provides stronger evidence.

Additionally researchers may collect data over a short or long time. In *cross-sectional* studies researchers collect data at a single point in time or at points close together, such as immediately before and after a treatment. In *longitudinal* studies, however, investigators collect data multiple times over a long time, sometimes decades, either from the same subjects (*panel study*) or from different subjects drawn from the larger population (*trend study*). Think of a cross-sectional study as analogous to a still photograph and a longitudinal one as a multiframe movie.

2.1.2 Researcher Assumptions

Assumptions are ideas that are accepted as true without testing, and they are present in all studies. Every researcher operates within a paradigm (or worldview) that is a set of assumptions about reality, truth, and values. Assumptions are important because they affect both what investigators choose to study and how they study it. For example, all researchers studying diabetes assume that gaining knowledge about diabetes is worthwhile and that some methods of studying it work better than others. At the same time, some may be more interested in individuals' subjective experiences, while others focus on pathophysiology.

One of the below major paradigms fits your research idea. Identify it for insight into your own assumptions.

1. Positivists assume that reality is objective, measurable, and discoverable by an impartial researcher. Positivism underlies the scientific process of observing and measuring variables numerically. It's what most people think of when they hear the word "research." Examples include randomized drug trials examining laboratory values.
2. *Constructivists* assume that reality exists as experienced by the individual within that person's psychosocial-cultural-spiritual context. Investigators recognize that their own contexts affect their studies from beginning to end, and so they work to set aside (*bracket*) their self-identified biases. Constructivists seek to uncover emerging meanings of persons' experiences by analyzing qualitative data. An example is interviewing unhoused individuals to identify what a lack of shelter means to them.
3. Advocates assume that reality is centered in relationships between powerful oppressors and the marginalized oppressed. Thus, the primary aim of advocacy-based research is to empower the oppressed, for example by including participants as coresearchers.

2.2   What Is Not Research?

Evidence-based practice (EBP) and quality improvement (QI) are not research. EBP and QI are about using existing knowledge, while research is about discovery (Fig. 2.2). EBP translates research and non-research evidence into best practices, and QI uses local data to make incremental practice changes and monitor outcomes.

Research, EBP, and QI projects are sometimes not easily differentiated because all three require problem identification, protecting subjects, and data collection and analysis. *Evidence-informed QI* (EBQI) further blurs lines. Some healthcare sites require IRB review of QI and EBP with an abbreviated protocol template. Using regulatory definitions, the IRB is the final arbiter of whether your project is or is not research, regardless of how you label it. When in doubt about whether your project needs IRB review, consult the IRB, submit the project, and follow IRB feedback.

> **Alert!** Some journals publish only IRB-reviewed QI and EBP. Because IRBs oversee research, getting post-project approval is difficult to impossible. The IRB may be willing to investigate a late application, but if they find that your project required their approval, then you are in violation of US federal rules.

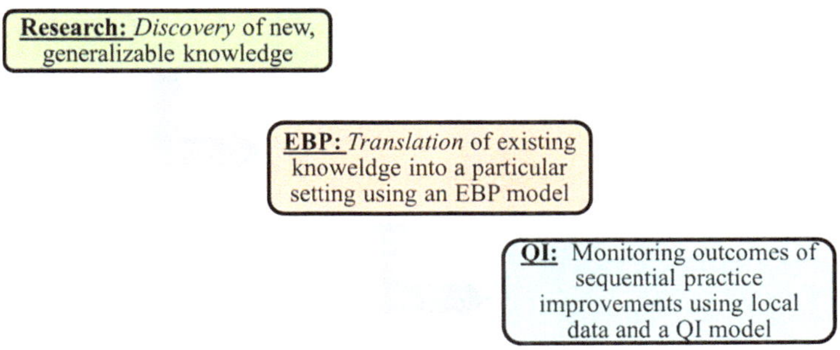

Research: *Discovery* of new, generalizable knowledge

EBP: *Translation* of existing knoweldge into a particular setting using an EBP model

QI: Monitoring outcomes of sequential practice improvements using local data and a QI model

Fig. 2.2   Research-EBP-QI relationships

2.2.1 Evidence-Based Practice (EBP)

EBP includes three elements: Evidence, clinician judgment, and preferences/values of patients and their families. EBP models outline similar steps summarized in Box 2.1. In EBP projects an individual or team adapts or adopts best practices for use in a particular setting and measures outcomes. An example is collecting data both before and after implementing a best practice on an entire unit.

Box 2.1 EBP Steps

1. Articulate the clinical problem.
2. Find and critique related research and non-research evidence.
3. Synthesize that evidence into site-specific, best practice recommendations.
4. Gain buy-in from *stakeholders*—those individuals or groups affected by the project.
5. Submit protocol for IRB review and follow their directives.
6. Implement the evidence-based practice change.
7. Collect and analyze outcome data.
8. Disseminate results to stakeholders and beyond.
9. Consolidate, adjust, and monitor the practice change as needed.

2.2.2 Quality Improvement (QI)

QI is a systematic process that typically uses ongoing rapid cycles of Plan-Do-Study-Act (PDSA) in order to guide incremental improvements in local care (Fig. 2.3). Steps are to Plan (identify an opportunity to improve practice), Do (enact the change), Study (measure and interpret outcomes), and Act (consolidate, modify, or abandon the change). QI projects may be based on a combination of local facility data, clinical observations, and scientific evidence. Project leaders consult with their QI departments.

Next step: Choosing an overall research plan

Fig. 2.3 Plan-Do-
Study Act model

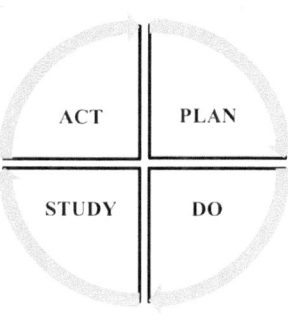

The Big Picture: Experiment vs. Non-Experiment

3

Key Points
- *An overall research design guides planning of study procedures.*
- *The two categories of overall design are experimental and nonexperimental.*
- *Experiments test researcher-manipulated interventions; non-experiments do not.*
- *Some unique healthcare-related design subtypes are mixed methods, methodological, ideological, and historical.*
- *The relationship between theory and research is a dynamic cycle.*

A research design provides overall study structure. Each design is like the framing of a house during construction. Just as a house frame provides structure and limits to walls, floors, and ceilings, so a research design provides structure and limits to a host of procedures. Different framing results in different houses, and different research designs result in different study methods.

Clinical research designs fall into two main categories: Experiments and non-experiments. Experiments test researcher-manipulated interventions; non-experiments do not. Non-experiments include surveys and observation studies.

Choose the design that fits your study purpose. To do this, first make sure your purpose is clear by completing this sentence: "The purpose of this study is…." Keep it brief, but specific, including the

© The Author(s), under exclusive license to Springer Nature Switzerland AG 2025
M. E. F. Highfield, *Doing Research*,
https://doi.org/10.1007/978-3-031-79044-7_3

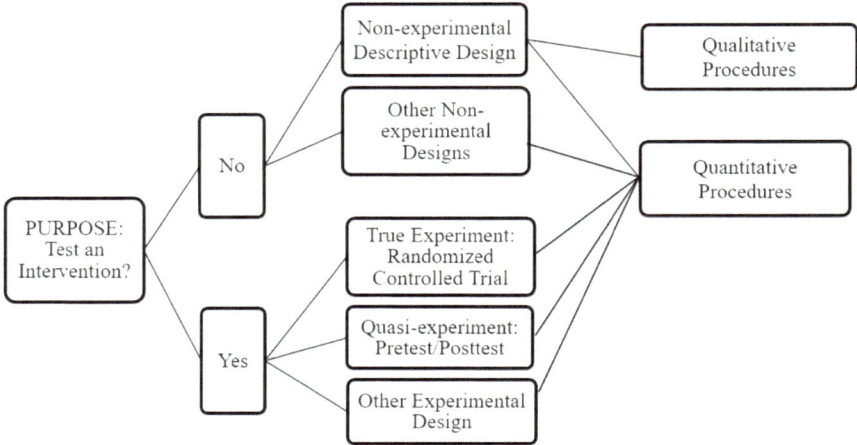

Fig. 3.1 Choosing a study design

who and what of your project. For example, "The purpose of this study is to describe NICU RNs' job satisfaction," or "The purpose is to test the effect of music listening on postoperative pain." Then select an appropriate design using Fig. 3.1 and the descriptions that follow.

> **Tip.** After reading below, record on the Protocol Worksheet the purpose and design that best fit your ideas. You can always modify it after your literature review.

3.1   Non-Experiments

3.1.1 Descriptive Studies

When little is known about a topic, researchers first describe it. Descriptive studies answer questions like "What are characteristics of [X]," "How often and under what circumstances does [X] occur," and so on.

Descriptive researchers use either quantitative and/or qualitative procedures (Box 3.1). Quantitative researchers ask questions that can be answered with numerical data and statistical analysis, such as "How long do staff wash their hands before patient contact?" Observers may measure handwashing minutes per contact, then calculate average minutes. In contrast, qualitative researchers collect and analyze narratives and documents in order to gain in-depth understanding of one variable. Data are analyzed using critical reflection, not statistics. For example, researchers might answer, "What are the experiences of first-time fathers?" by looking for common themes in transcribed interviews.

Box 3.1 Quantitative vs. Qualitative Procedures

	Quantitative	Qualitative
Data type	Numerical	Nonnumerical
Data analysis	Statistical	Examining & reexamining data to find patterns and meanings
Related design	Non-experiments or experiments	Descriptive non-experiments
Setting	Researcher-controlled	Natural, uncontrolled
Data collection procedures	Fixed in advance: Researcher-controlled with high structure	Flexible: Researchers observe how things unfold naturally
Researcher involvement	Short or long engagement with subjects by an objective research "outsider"	Intense, lengthy engagement with informants by a subjective researcher
Sampling	Predetermined size; ideally a random sample representing a larger population	No predetermined size; sampling may continue until no new information emerges (*data saturation*); usually a nonrandom sample who can describe their experiences
Instrument	High structure, such as a questionnaire or checklist	Low structure, such as interviews with *researcher-as-instrument*
Analysis timing	All data are collected and analyzed at single time point(s)	Data may be analyzed as they are collected (*constant comparison*)

(continued)

Box 3.1 (continued)

	Quantitative	Qualitative
Results	Population characteristics: Reports summarize all data	Individual characteristics: Reports use examples of data
Generalizability	Often	Rarely; possible *transferability*
Coinvestigators	Statistician & colleagues	Informants & colleagues
View of reality	Reductionist; reality as separate bits	Wholistic, integrated
View of persons	Objects to whom things are done	Subjects who do things
Assumptions	Positivist	Constructivist

Common qualitative design subtypes are in Box 3.2. These are most valuable in creating understanding of one phenomenon and raising questions for future study. Their purpose is descriptive.

Box 3.2 Qualitative Designs

Design	Focus	Example	Origin
Case study/case series	A single event or phenomenon in a particular time & place; a case series includes up to four cases	Report on one patient with food-medication interaction	Social science
Ethnography	Culture or subculture characteristics, such as meanings, communications, & mores	Staff culture of safety in the emergency room	Anthropology
Grounded theory	The basic social process (BSP) of how participants confront a social problem; an "-ing" word often names the process	"Fearing to comfort:… constraints to opioid use in hospice care" [1]	Sociology

(continued)

Box 3.2 (continued)

Design	Focus	Example	Origin
Narrative	Stories about the meaning of & experiences with a phenomenon or event	First-hand accounts of admitting family members to a memory care facility	Literary critique; History; Social science
Phenomenology	The essence of informants' "lived experiences" of an event or situation; what they experienced & how	The lived experience of new registered nurse graduates in critical care	Philosophy & psychology

Alert! All qualitative studies are descriptive, but not all descriptive studies are qualitative.

3.1.2 Correlation Studies

Correlation studies identify whether changes in one or more variable(s) are statistically related to changes in one or more others. Investigators explore whether different variables increase or decrease in the same or opposite directions at the same time. Correlation researchers answer questions like, "Are changes in [variable X] and in [variable Y] related?" or test hypotheses like, "As [variable X] increases, [variable Y] decreases."

Alert! Correlation is not causation.

Just because two variables are related does not mean that one causes change in the other. Like chickens and eggs, no one can say which came first. For example, when researchers find that more years of practice are associated with higher job satisfaction, it may be that longer practice caused more satisfaction, or that satisfaction caused longer practice, or that a third variable like workplace environment created change in both.

3.1.3 Cohort & Case-Controlled Studies

In cohort and case-controlled studies, investigators observe populations over an extended time—sometimes years. Both designs focus on
identifying statistical associations between a potential health risk and
its effects. Both are useful because it is unethical for researchers to
expose individuals to disease or disability. Instead they observe natural   occurrences.   Neither   design   has   a   researcher-controlled
intervention.

Cohort and case-controlled methods also differ. Usually cohort
studies are prospective, and case controlled studies retrospective. A
cohort study identifies emerging health trends among subjects after
their exposure to an already existing possible cause. This is called *ex
post facto* (after the fact) research. An example is studying the inci-
dence of lung disease among marijuana smokers. In contrast, a case-
controlled study starts with a group of those exhibiting health effects
(cases) and a group who does not (controls), and then describes exposure of both to an earlier potential cause. An example is whether cases
with type 2 diabetes and controls without it were bottle fed as infants.

3.2   Experiments

Experiments test whether researcher-controlled interventions change
outcomes. The intervention is the cause or *independent variable*. The
outcome is the effect or *dependent variable* because its variation
depends on changes in the intervention. Experiments use hypotheses,
quantitative data, and statistical analysis.

> **Alert!** No variable is inherently a cause/independent or effect/
> dependent one. The same variable could be causative in one
> study and the outcome in another.

An example of a hypothesis and its variables is, "Bowel function
returns more quickly among post-operative patients who chew gum
than among post-operative patients who don't chew gum." In this
case, researchers manipulate the intervention (cause/independent
variable) of gum chewing so that it is present for some patients and

Fig. 3.2 Example of study & extraneous variables

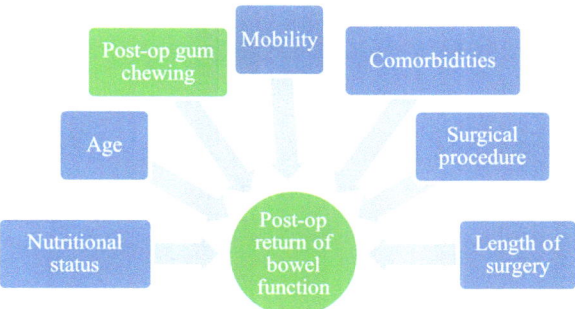

absent for others, and then they measure bowel function return (effect/dependent variable). Statistical tests compare outcomes for gum-chewers versus non-gum-chewers to see if differences between the two groups are greater than would happen by chance alone.

Experimental researchers must also control *extraneous variables* that interfere with studying their hypotheses. Continuing with the gum-chewing example, Fig. 3.2 shows the researcher-hypothesized cause and effect in green alongside extraneous variables in blue. In order to isolate the effect of gum chewing on bowel function, researchers must control the "blue" variables so they do not become alternative explanations for bowel function return (*rival hypotheses*). A rival hypothesis example is, "Mobility or age [not gum chewing] improved bowel function return."

> **Tip.** Use both your experience and literature to identify extraneous variables that might affect results.

Investigators use three methods to control extraneous variables. First, they might turn extraneous variables into study variables by including them in hypotheses. In the Fig. 3.2 example investigators might write a hypothesis that includes all "blue" and "green" causative variables, and then statistically analyze how much each one contributes to bowel function return.

Second, researchers might recruit a sample that is the same (*homogenous*) in age, nutritional status, mobility, and so on. This turns extraneous variables into *constants* that don't vary and so can't interfere with results. Finally others might include a description of extraneous variables in sample demographics and let readers judge how well the sample matches their own patients. Investigators may use different options for different extraneous variables in the same study.

> **Alert!** In reality you can neither anticipate nor control all extraneous variables. Control those likely to have a substantial influence on outcomes.

3.2.1 Randomized Controlled Trials

Randomized controlled trials (RCTs) are true experiments that minimize rival hypotheses. Their three elements are randomization, a control group, and an intervention. Participants are randomly assigned (*randomized*) to either experimental or control groups, and then the experimental group receives a new intervention while the control group often receives standard therapy. RCTs may use more than two groups. Group outcomes are compared in what is called a *between group trial* because each group contains different subjects. For example, investigators might assign each ovarian cancer patient in their clinic to either standard therapy or a novel one and then compare outcomes of intra-treatment and posttreatment symptoms, quality of life, and disease progression.

3.2.2 Quasi-Experiments

Quasi-experiments test an intervention but lack either randomization and/or a control group. A *pretest/posttest* is perhaps the most common type. Pretest/posttest *within group trials* compare the same subjects' pre-intervention data with their post-intervention data; pre-intervention measurements are equivalent to control group outcomes. In other words, subjects serve as their own controls. Statistical analysis compares the before and after average group scores (*unpaired data*) or the before and after scores of individuals (*paired data*). Paired analysis is more precise.

Nonequivalent control group design is another type of quasi-experiment. It is used when randomization is impossible and the alternative is not to study a topic at all. For example, when comparing practices of staff with associate degrees versus baccalaureate degrees, researchers cannot randomize students to schools and must assume that people choosing different degree programs are already not alike (nonequivalent). This means that something other than degree might affect practice—a rival hypothesis!

3.2.3 Selected Other Experiments

Posttest only, cross-over, and factorial designs are just three other experimental subtypes. *Posttest only studies* measure only post-intervention outcomes without baseline data or a control group. That makes them closer to descriptive studies and far from RCTs.

In *cross-over designs* all randomized subjects receive all interventions, thus allowing researchers to measure changes both within and between groups. An example is randomizing participants into two groups with each group receiving either naturopathic remedies or standard medication, measuring outcomes, and then putting both groups through a "palette-cleansing" wash out period. After that investigators give each group the alternative intervention and measure outcomes again.

Finally, in *factorial designs* numerous subjects are randomized into at least four groups, and each group receives a different combination of interventions. This requires many subjects! In the Table 3.1 example, researchers identify both *main effects* of the treatment factors (nicotine vs. lobelia) and the *interaction effects* of those same factors plus levels of weekly vs. monthly counseling. Compared outcomes are the number of smokers within each group who quit.

Table 3.1 Factorial design: fictional smoking cessation intervention study ($N = 120$)

	Weekly counseling	Monthly counseling
Medication treatment: Nicotine patch	Group 1 ($n = 30$)	Group 3 ($n = 30$)
Naturopathic treatment: Lobelia	Group 2 ($n = 30$)	Group 4 ($n = 30$)

3.3   Mixed Methods Designs

Mixed methods (MM) research provides a more complete picture of reality by analyzing complementary quantitative and qualitative data together in a single study. A clinical analogy for MM research is asking patients both to rate their pain numerically on a 0–10 scale and to describe its non-numerical character, location, and severity. An MM study may be primarily an experiment, a non-experiment, or a combination.

Common MM subtypes are in Box 3.3. In *concurrent* (*convergent*) *designs* investigators collect all quantitative and qualitative data at the same time, while in *sequential designs* they collect one type of data before the other. In sequential MM, researchers give more weight to whatever data were collected first. In *triangulated MM*, however, all data receive equal weight, while in *embedded designs*, such as a large RCT in which only a few participants are interviewed, the smaller data subset receives less weight.

Box 3.3 Mixed Methods Designs

Design	Priority weighted data
Concurrent data collection	
• Triangulation	All data equally weighted
• Embedded	Main study data
Sequential data collection	
• Exploratory	Qualitative data
• Explanatory	Quantitative data

3.4   Methodological Research

Methodological research focuses on how to study a topic, not on the topic itself. The aim is to improve research methods. Methodological investigators may use experiments and non-experiments to develop new data collection tools or to test study procedures. An example of tool development is creating a new fall risk checklist by using patient fall data, observations, literature review, expert opinion, and statistics to establish the checklist's reliability (consistency) and validity (accuracy). (See Chap. 8 for more on tools.) Another example of methodological research imbedded in many larger studies is a *pilot study*.

A pilot study is a small-scale test of planned study procedures to make sure they work well before using them in a full-scale investigation; pilots do not provide preliminary research answers.

3.5   Ideological Research

What differentiates ideological research is its emphasis on empowering oppressed groups rather than on knowledge discovery. Its origins are Marxist political theory with advocacy assumptions. Investigators use nonexperimental and experimental designs and methods in order to critique society, raise awareness, and inspire social action. Three subtype examples are *community-based participatory action research* that engages informants as coinvestigators, *feminist research* that seeks to empower women, and *critical theory research* that seeks to undermine oppressive societal structures.

3.6   Historical Research

Historians shed light on the present and future by critically examining the meaning of past events. They are not mere story-tellers. Their data are *primary sources* from the time being studied and *secondary sources* that are later, filtered information. For example, Florence Nightingale's letters are a primary source, while a twentieth century book about her is a secondary one. More weight is given to primary sources, but no source is accepted without question and without comparison to other information. Neither primary nor secondary sources contain complete, objective information, and either may contain factual errors. Historians analyze their primary and secondary sources within the sources' original historical context. Reliance on past data limits the questions that historians can answer.

3.7   Postscript on Research, Practice, & Theory

Theories about effective clinical practices are built, tested, and revised through research, for example germ theory and handwashing. Specifically non-experiments build theory and experiments test theory in a continuous cycle. Non-experiments describe and connect information about a topic until an understanding of the whole subject emerges. This *inductive* process of moving from specific research findings to general theory is analogous to assembling jigsaw pieces into relationship with each other until we see the complete picture (theory). Then researchers use *deductive* logic to hypothesize and experimentally test how well that theory explains and predicts clinical outcomes. If the theory explains and predicts well, testing continues in new situations. If it explains and predicts poorly, we revise the theory then test again.

Next steps: Some practical matters

Reference

1. Zerwekh J, Riddell S, Richard J. Fearing to comfort: a grounded theory of constraints to opioid use in hospice care. J Hosp Palliat Nurs. 2002;4:83–90.

Make Practical Preparations

4

Key Points

- *Add design to your purpose statement.*
- *Draft a project title and at least one measurable hypothesis or question (H/Q).*
- *Identify institutional review board (IRB) requirements, forms, fees, and deadlines.*
- *Complete IRB-required ethics training.*
- *Engage stakeholders and identify research-site required procedures.*
- *Gather topic-related research and non-research literature.*
- *Artificial intelligence (AI) is currently unreliable for literature searches.*

4.1 Refine Study Purpose

Add research design to your purpose statement. Examples are: "The purpose of this *descriptive,* cross-sectional study is to identify public health staff job satisfaction;" or "The purpose of this *quasi-experiment* is to test the effect of lactation counselor support on breastfeeding duration."

For qualitative studies, consider this script: "The purpose of this_____(narrative, phenomenological, grounded theory, ethnographic, case) study is… to_____(understand? describe? develop? discover?) the_____[variable of interest]…for_____(the participants)

© The Author(s), under exclusive license to Springer Nature Switzerland AG 2025   23
M. E. F. Highfield, *Doing Research*,
https://doi.org/10.1007/978-3-031-79044-7_4

at _____(the site)." [1, p. 199] For example "The purpose of this phe-nomenological study is to describe the lived experiences of Black students in a top-tier medical school."

> **Tip.** Anything you write at this point is a draft, so don't let the perfect be the enemy of the good. Focus on getting your thoughts on paper.

4.2   Draft a Hypothesis or Question

Next, translate your broad purpose into measurable H/Qs that include study population and study variable(s). In qualitative studies the purpose may double as the research question. Otherwise the optional acronym PICOT (Population/problem, Intervention, Comparison to intervention, Outcome, Timing) may help (Box 4.1). PICOT is especially helpful to generate keywords for library searching.

Note that PICOT is a tool, not a rule. Thus, some use PICO without (T) or have more than one comparison group (C). Nonexperimental researchers may use only PIO or PEO (Population, Exposure to/ Involvement in a situation, and Outcome).

> **Tip.** If PICOT is more confusing than helpful, skip it. What you cannot skip is identifying your population and research variable(s).

After identifying your population and variable(s) incorporate them into an H/Q using optional Box 4.2 scripts. Hypothesize only when scientific literature suggests a relationship between variables. Otherwise ask a question. Hypotheses always appear in experiments, sometimes in correlation studies, and never in descriptive research.

Box 4.1 PICOT & Examples

PICOT	Non-experiment example	Experiment example
P = population in which you are interested or **problem** that needs solving; may include setting	Adults with new spinal cord injury admitted to the rehabilitation unit	
I = intervention [for non-experiments, substitute **I (involvement in)** or **E (exposure to)** something]	Status quo physical therapy (PT)	PT with therapy dogs
C = comparison to intervention group		PT without therapy dogs
O = outcome measured by data collection tool	Motivation to complete PT	
T = timing of measurements	On rehab admission	On rehab admission & again at discharge

Box 4.2 From PICOT to H/Q

Study design	H or Q	Script
Descriptive—Describes one variable at a time	Question	What is (O)___ among (P) ___ exposed to (I/E) ___?
Correlational—Asks whether changes in 2 or more variables are related	Question	Is there an association between exposure to (I/E)___and (O) ___ among (P) ____?
Correlational—Tests a predicted association between 2 or more variables	Hypothesis	(I/E) ___ is associated with [changes? increases? decreases?] in (O)___ among (P) ___ at (T) ___.
Experimental—Tests outcomes of a researcher-controlled intervention	Hypothesis	(P) ___ receiving (I) ___ will have [higher/lower/different] (O) ___ at (T) ___ than will (P) ___ receiving (C) ___ at (T) ___.

4.3   Draft Title

Your title is a mini-abstract that communicates who and what you are studying. Include population (P), intervention/exposure (I/E), outcome (O), and perhaps design. Avoid writing it as a question. This is a working draft to be refined after writing your full protocol.

Tip. Review titles of published research for examples.

4.4   Engage Stakeholders

Garner support from stakeholders, such as supervisors or facility researchers. No one affected by your project wants to be surprised. Moreover, an unaware stakeholder may unintentionally undercut your project. Brainstorm what each might want to know and identify their communication preferences (e.g., email, face-to-face). Act accordingly.

Active support from administrative and research stakeholders adds credibility and potential project champions. Share with them the topic, how your research addresses it, and anticipated project benefits. Describe resources you bring to the project, including clinical expertise, mentor, and any funds. Explain your timeline, welcome input, and if you need something from them, ask. If your plans are preliminary, keep stakeholders up-to-date. Remember that people are busy and resources tight. Some are happy for you to do a project as long as it demands little of them.

Tip: Aligning your project with institutional priorities is a good way to get stakeholder support.

Delineate any role and pay issues. Avoid mixing paid work with any unpaid research activities, and comply with facility policies. Also, if yours is a school project, contact the research-site person who manages university-facility affiliation agreements to identify relevant requirements.

A leader, researcher, or committee at the research site may need to sign off on the project before it goes to the IRB. Their input may also prevent time-consuming mistakes. When possible invite your mentor to accompany you to any committee meetings to help with technical research issues, but be prepared to explain your own project. Permission from a unit manager is not enough to conduct a study.

4.5   Identify IRB Requirements

Before conducting a study, you need IRB approval of your protocol. Think of the IRB as your friend: It protects you, the institution, and your participants by making sure that your research plans are ethical and legal. All US IRBs follow the same federal regulations, although procedures vary.

Alert! Never contact subjects or begin any part of your study—no matter how seemingly harmless—until you receive written IRB authorization.

Identify IRB forms, fees, and deadlines in your university and/or the research site. Remember to write your protocol using the relevant IRB template in order to facilitate swift approval. If no template exists, use this book's Protocol Worksheet and Chaps. 5, 6, 7, 8 and 9 as protocol guides. Finally, at the research-site be prepared to pay an IRB review fee if you are an outsider or have grant funding; unfunded students and employees may be exempt. Ascertain any review fees before investing time in a project.

Students, including facility employees, should generally obtain IRB approval first from their university and then from the research site. Others need only the latter.

Alert! You must have IRB approval, but the research site is not required to have an IRB.

Many healthcare facilities don't have an IRB. Some affiliate with an outside one, or you can ask a university or other IRB to review your project. They may, however, refuse or charge a fee.

No IRB approval is required for administrative projects, evaluation of educational programs, course exams, single case studies, and most oral histories or biographies. Nonetheless, consult the IRB website for whether your project needs review, and contact them about anything confusing. The IRB itself may need to review your project to verify exemption in writing, such as with oral histories. Keep copies of IRB communications.

4.6   Take Ethics Training

IRBs require proof of ethics training, usually from either CITI (Collaborative Institutional Training Initiative) or US NIH (National Institutes of Health) Human Research Protection Foundational Training. Both educational programs are online and self-paced. If the IRB requires CITI training, log in through your institution's link to avoid fees.

Allow several hours for initial training. You may need to complete only some CITI or NIH modules, so consult your mentor. CITI training documentation is transferable to other facilities and requires renewal refresher modules every few years. Maintain current ethics training throughout a project.

4.7   Gather Literature

Conduct a thorough topic-related search of the literature. Make friends with the librarian as an information expert who can search for you. Then you can spend more time reading and writing a summary. Moreover, librarian-assisted searches have higher credibility. (See Appendix A for basics of doing your own search.)

To start a search, share with the librarian your H/Q and any on-target research articles that you already located. Additionally ask the librarian to include *grey literature*: Credible documents outside peer-reviewed publications, such as government reports. The librarian then sorts through millions of publications and presents you with a list of topic-related titles and abstracts, as well as search terms and databases used. Always thank the librarian, and never hesitate to ask for more help.

Tip. On the Protocol Worksheet, record search terms and databases used. You'll want this for your final dissemination report or to refine your search.

Obtain full text copies of relevant articles; never rely on abstracts. Print and date hard copies of any webpage content because websites vanish and change. Finally, copy and paste authors, dates, titles or URLs of publications to create a draft protocol reference list. Worry about format later.

A search may identify too many or too few articles. If you find thousands, narrow your search terms, or start with the most current and strongest evidence and then stop when you begin reading no new information. If, however, you locate very few, then ask the librarian to widen the search. Even one article may be enough to design a safe, ethical, and feasible project that includes rigorous outcome measures [2].

Alert! Artificial intelligence (AI) is currently unreliable for literature searches.

Do not use rapidly evolving AI to search literature. ChatGPT, for example, is not linked to library healthcare databases, so you must independently check AI-generated sources to see if they exist. ChatGPT creates fake authors, titles, or research findings and mixes these with real ones. If using AI, verify information and inform readers that you used AI. A librarian can help with how AI can be used if at all.

Next step: Explain why your study is important

References

1. Creswell JW, Poth C. Qualitative inquiry and research design: choosing among five approaches. 4th ed. Los Angeles: Sage; 2018.
2. Deets C. When is enough, enough? J Prof Nurs. 1998;14:196.

Synthesize Literature

5

Key Points
- *Use literature to document the background and significance of your topic.*
- *Evaluate both the strength and quality of each research article.*
- *For quantitative studies define your study variables, and describe the relationships between them, ideally using an established theory or framework.*
- *Identify the gap in knowledge that your study fills.*

Read your retrieved literature to build topic-related expertise, define key variables, identify useful research procedures, and even get a head start on final dissemination. This chapter will help you evaluate, summarize, and synthesize existing research in order to write the background and significance protocol section.

The background and significance section summarizes current literature. Significance is the problem's impact and prevalence, while background contains what we know and don't know about the topic. If almost no literature exists, qualitative research may be warranted.

> **Tip.** Models for writing background and significance are in the introductory sections of published research on your topic. Be careful not to plagiarize.

© The Author(s), under exclusive license to Springer Nature Switzerland AG 2025   31
M. E. F. Highfield, *Doing Research*,
https://doi.org/10.1007/978-3-031-79044-7_5

5.1   Use Best Evidence

Use the highest quality, strongest research available to write background and significance. Quality is how meticulously investigators adhered to scientific methods (Sect. 5.2.2), and strength is based on design. Figure 5.1 illustrates the strongest research designs at the pyramid top and the weakest at its base. The pyramid assumes that quantitative cause-and-effect research best reflects reality—a positivist approach.

If you find a top-of-pyramid meta-analysis, systematic review, or EB clinical guideline, then much is known about your topic. These are generalizable evidence, so you can rely heavily on them for writing background and significance. Otherwise rely on the strongest evidence you do find.

If you find only evidence near the pyramid base, then we know little. In such cases, where evidence is low-level, scant, or conflicting, consider adding your personal observations to background as "anecdotal evidence." If you do this, do not assume that your casual observations represent anyone else anywhere else; they can raise important questions, but are not generalizable.

Also design (or redesign) your project to build on existing research. This means that if you find only expert opinions about your topic, then a non-experiment is the next logical step. An intervention study might be premature.

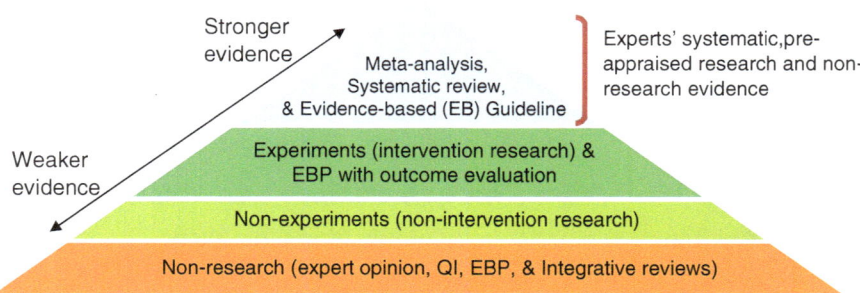

Fig. 5.1 Strength of evidence overview. (See Box 5.1 for ranked research designs within each level.)

Alert! The pyramid is a guide, and rankings assume that all projects are equally well-done. A high quality study that is low on the pyramid can be stronger evidence than a low quality study that is higher. *Caveat emptor.*

5.2 Organize, Read, Write

Writing background and significance requires converting a stack of articles into a coherent, orderly protocol section. One way to do this is first to organize articles by strength, then read them for quality and content, and finally write. As with PICOT, these three steps are a tool, not a rule; use part, all, or none.

5.2.1 Step 1: Organize

Separate articles into two stacks: Research and non-research. Any published protocols are non-research because they are plans only, not completed studies. Second, order the research articles from strongest to weakest designs (Box 5.1). The design is in the title, abstract, or methods/procedures. Third, number research then non-research articles consecutively, and use those numbers as draft footnotes to cite as you write.

Box 5.1 Strength of Specific Designs: Strongest to Weakest

Design	Description
Meta-analysis	*Statistical synthesis* of findings from all relevant *quantitative studies* into one larger study using transparent, published, standardized, systematic methods.
Systematic review	*Nonstatistical integration* of findings from *all relevant studies using* transparent, published, standardized, systematic methods (e.g., Cochrane Collaboration). Systematic reviews of RCTs are stronger than systematic reviews of correlational studies which are stronger than systematic reviews of descriptive studies.

(continued)

Box 5.1 (continued)

Design	Description
EB clinical guideline	*Nonstatistical*, methodical, transparent integration of *research and non-research findings* into *practice recommendations.* EB guidelines use research, but are not research themselves.
Randomized controlled trial (RCT)	[See Chap. 3]
Quasi-experiment	[See Chap. 3]
Evidence-based practice (EBP)	EBP project with measured outcomes
Correlational study	[See Chap. 3]
Descriptive quantitative study[a]	[See Chap. 3]
Meta-synthesis	*Nonstatistical synthesis* of findings from multiple *qualitative studies* using a published, transparent, methodical process.
Case controlled study	[See Chap. 3]
Cohort study	[See Chap. 3]
Descriptive qualitative study	[See Chap. 3]

Note: Generalizability from RCT down depends on scientific quality (rigor) of the particular study. *Transferability* of qualitative studies corresponds to quantitative generalizability.

[a]QI is sometimes ranked as equivalent in strength to a descriptive quantitative study.

Alert! Beware similar sounding names:

1. *Systematic reviews* critique all relevant research to establish best clinical practices.
2. *Scoping reviews* critique all relevant research to overview the state of the science [1].
3. *Integrative reviews* are expert opinion using limited, author-selected literature.
4. *EB clinical guidelines* synthesize all research and non-research to identify best practices.
5. *EBP projects* apply best practices in a particular setting and evaluate outcomes.

5.2.2 Step 2: Read & Assess Quality

First read the non-research articles for an overview, then move on to research. Starting with the strongest research, review abstract, tables, and figures. Next underline key information (Box 5.2), and finally read the article beginning to end. Re-read as needed. Repeat this process with each article, and consult your mentor about anything you don't understand.

Box 5.2 Key Study Information

Article section	What to underline
Title & Abstract	• Main variable(s)
	• Population
Introduction/Literature review/Background	• Problem statement (often in first 1–2 sentences)
	• Background (summarized in topic sentences)
	• H/Qs (often the last 1–2 sentences)
Methods/Procedures	• Research design (often in first sentences)
	• Sample, including who can and cannot be in the study
	• Sampling method: random or nonrandom
	• Setting
Results/Findings	• Only findings related to your own purpose and H/Q
Limitations	• Generalizability or transferability of results
Discussion/Implications	• Meaning of outcomes (often topic sentences)

Tip. Instead of underlining, consider creating an optional summary table of evidence, like the one at https://www.ncbi.nlm.nih.gov/books/NBK2659/table/ch7.t1/.

Evaluate each study's quality (*rigor*) using applicable quantitative (Box 5.3) or qualitative criteria (Box 5.4). Rate each study's quality on a 1–3 scale: (1) *acceptable* with no major issues, (2) *limited* with many or major flaws, or (3) *unacceptable* when executed so poorly that you have little confidence in its findings. Drop those rated "3" from consideration. Alternatively use a quality rating scale from your professional organization or a credible EBP model, like Johns Hopkins' [2].

Alert! Never accept research findings only because you like them. Never reject findings only because you don't.

Box 5.3 Quantitative Study Rigor

Criteria	Definition	Supportive article content
Internal study validity	*Accurate answers* to H/Qs: Confidence that the independent variable (intervention) is what changed outcomes	Rigorous procedures* controlled extraneous variables & answered well-articulated H/Qs
External study validity	*Generalizability*: Confidence that findings are applicable to the larger population	*Representativeness* of sample and rigorous procedures

*Sampling, intervention, measurement, and analysis.

Box 5.4 Qualitative Study Rigor

Criteria	Definition	Supportive article content
Dependability	How likely is it that others would find similar results *later if replicated*?	Detailed descriptions; procedure audit
Confirmability	How likely is it that a *different researcher* would have found the same results?	Researcher journaling; *bracketing* (*reflexivity*)
Credibility	How well do findings *represent reality*?	*Member checks*; *triangulation*; *prolonged engagement*
Transferability	How *similar* are study setting & subjects to other settings & subjects?	Detailed (*thick*) description of setting and informants

5.2.3 Step 3: Write

Don't wait for a block of time. Don't talk instead of writing. Make daily, even tiny writing appointments with yourself. Set a timer for 5–10 minutes, reset it if productive, and break every 30–60 minutes to stretch and hydrate. Consider linking your new writing habit to an existing habit like morning coffee [3].

> **Tip.** For group writing support join a local Shut Up and Write event (https://shutupwrite.com), or make a pact with like-minded colleagues.

Write in three stages: Prewrite (draft), write, and rewrite (edit). Start by reviewing your study purpose and H/Qs, then prewrite by jotting down important phrases, words, or sketches.

Brainstorm, free write, journal, or make lists. Don't worry about complete sentences. Use circles or arrows to connect ideas, and start writing in the middle or end if easier. Online prewriting suggestions abound.

> **Alert!** Always cite as you write, no matter how rushed you feel. Use your numbering on articles as interim, shorthand footnotes.

Use underlined article information to summarize each study including sample, setting, design, and results relevant to your purpose and H/Qs. Skip non-related results. For example, if your own project is about music and pain a fictitious example is: "Sikes et al. pre/post study: 289-bed, Magnet, teaching hospital; 193 patients reported less pain after 15 minutes of nature sounds music (p = .03)." If study findings conflict, document author explanations or your ideas, such as different samples or data collection tools.

Alert! Never use article content as summarized by someone else. Always write from the original publication.

Draft your significance and background based on any top-of-pyramid evidence (earlier Fig. 5.1). Then add un-included, more recent studies that support or refute it. Alternatively if evidence is scant summarize it, and assure readers that your search was thorough by recording search terms, databases, and librarian assistance.

An example prewrite for significance and background is: "Burnout is high among U.S. critical care staff [references]. Burnout is defined as_____according to_____framework/theory [reference]. Burnout is important to resolve because it produces negative outcomes of_____ [references]. Sources of staff burnout include_____[references]. Potential solutions are_____ [references]. What we don't know is_____."

Tip. Numerous literature review templates are at https://templatelab.com/literature-review/

After prewriting, write. Organize your prewrite draft into an introduction, main points, and conclusion using complete sentences and paragraphs. In the introduction state the problem and its frequency and impact in one to five sentences. Then for main points, group your research article summaries thematically or chronologically. Use transition words like "since [year/event]," "first," "second," "additionally," "moreover," or "lastly." Explain conflicting findings. Finally in a conclusion summarize in one to five sentences what is known and not known.

Next rewrite (edit) for style and detail. Topic sentences should make an orderly line of reasoning by themselves. If they don't, rearrange, add, or subtract information. Sentences in each paragraph should relate to the topic sentence. To catch other mistakes, read your paper aloud to yourself or use your word processing software "read aloud" or "accessibility" function. Electronically check spelling and grammar, and format references. Ask a colleague to read your work for clarity. Lastly, make sure your background and significance section addresses all IRB-required information.

> **Alert!** Don't allow bad writing to sabotage a good project. Prewriting, writing, and rewriting are useful throughout protocol development and dissemination.

5.3   Definitions & Framework

In the background for a quantitative study devote at least a paragraph to the framework or theory that defines your variables and specifies relationships between them. Using a separate "Framework" subheading may make this easier. The framework or theory describes, explains, or makes predictions about your topic. Example frameworks are human physiology, Kübler-Ross's stages of grief, teaching-learning theories, and gate control pain theory.

> **Alert!** Qualitative investigators use the term "framework" differently to refer to their design, such as ethnography or case study.

Selecting a quantitative study framework is far easier and more practical than it may sound. First, your research and non-research articles often describe topic-related frameworks. Adopting one of those elevates your project to a whole new scientific level: Your results are easily compared with others'.

Additionally the framework defines your outcome variable(s) in two ways. First, it provides an abstract, dictionary-type *conceptual definition*, and second it may offer a concrete, measurable *operational definition* in the form of a data collection tool. For example, Ellison and Paloutzian conceptually defined spiritual quality of life (QOL) as a subjective sense of both religious and existential well-being. They then operationally defined spiritual QOL as their Spiritual Well-Being Scale that quantifies self-reported religious and existential well-being as a score [4].

> **Tip.** If you find a relevant data collection tool first, then you can work backwards to find its framework in a tool manual or methodological study.

For some topics conceptual and operational definitions don't exist. In that case plan qualitative, theory-building research in order to describe variables and the relationships between them. At other times only methodological research is needed to develop an instrument (operational definition) that measures a conceptually defined variable.

Next step: Plan step-by-step procedures

References

1. Munn Z, Peters MDJ, Stern C, Tufanaru C, McArthur A, Aromataris E. Systematic review or scoping review? Guidance for authors when choosing between a systematic or scoping review approach. BMC Med Res Methodol. 2018;18:1–7.
2. Dang D, Dearholt S, Bissett K, Ascenzi J, Whalen M. Johns Hopkins evidence-based practice for nurses and healthcare professionals: model and guidelines. 4th ed. Sigma Theta Tau International; 2022. https://www.hopkinsmedicine.org/evidence-based-practice/model-tools. Accessed 4 October 2024.
3. Clear J. Atomic habits: an easy & proven way to build good habits & break bad ones. New York: Penguin; 2018.
4. Ellison RF, Paloutzian CW (1991–2021). Manual for the spiritual well-being scale. https://www.westmont.edu/sites/default/files/users/user401/SWBS%20Manual%202.0_0.pdf. Accessed 15 March 2024.

Design Rigorous Procedures

6

Key Points
- *Before writing procedures, refine hypotheses/questions (H/Qs) one more time in light of reviewed literature.*
- *Consider replicating others' studies using their H/Qs and procedures in part or whole.*
- *Plan rigorous procedures that minimize threats to study accuracy (validity).*
- *To plan ethical and feasible procedures consider risks, resources, and readiness.*

The best procedures are those likely to yield accurate answers to clearly stated H/Qs. Thus, your plans for sampling, any intervention, instrument(s), and data collection and analysis must be scientifically rigorous, minimize threats to study accuracy, and be ethical yet feasible within your time and budget.

6.1 Refine Hypotheses or Research Questions

Before writing procedures, revise, add to, or subtract from your H/Qs as needed based on your newly acquired, literature-based knowledge. Typically quantitative studies have two to five H/Qs, and a qualitative

© The Author(s), under exclusive license to Springer Nature Switzerland AG 2025
M. E. F. Highfield, *Doing Research*,
https://doi.org/10.1007/978-3-031-79044-7_6

study one. Depending on study design you may write only questions, only hypotheses, or a combination. Remember to name the population, any intervention, and outcome variable(s) in each.

Tip. Obtain a model for your protocol by asking your mentor for an existing IRB-approved one that uses your same research design (e.g., pretest/posttest). You don't have to follow it exactly.

6.1.1 Quantitative Hypotheses & Questions

Quantitative studies may answer questions or test hypotheses. A question may start with "What is…" or "Is there a relationship between…," while a hypothesis asserts a testable statement about variable relationships. Only experimental hypotheses should use words like "cause," "improve," "affect" or their synonyms, while correlational hypotheses use phrases like "associated with."

Alert! A hypothesis may be worded as a declaration or a question. A predicted relationship between variables is what makes it a hypothesis—not the punctuation mark.

Your H/Qs will be either simple or complex (Box 6.1), as well as nondirectional or directional. When we know little, nondirectional H/Qs suggest neutrally that one variable "affects" or "is related to" another. When we know more, directional H/Qs specify either a *positive relationship* in which variables rise and fall together or an *inverse relationship* in which one variable goes up as the other goes down. Directional H/Qs use words like "increase," "decrease," and "enhance."

Box 6.1 Simple vs. Complex Hypotheses & Questions

Experimental hypotheses

- Simple   Hypothesis with only one cause and one effect variable
- Complex   Hypothesis with more than one cause and/or more than one effect variable

Correlational H/Qs

- Simple   H/Q examining an association between two variables
- Complex   H/Q examining an association between more than two variables

Two other sometimes confusing types of hypotheses are null and rival ones. First, a null hypothesis is used only for statistical purposes and is never stated in a protocol or final report. Each stated research hypotheses has a corollary null (statistical) one, and so while your research hypothesis asserts that experimental and control group outcomes will differ, the null states that they will be the same. Statistics are then used to disprove the null. Second, a rival hypothesis is that an extraneous variable not the researcher-controlled intervention created results.

6.1.2 Qualitative Questions

Qualitative studies answer questions that are linked to design, so much so that study purpose may double as the research question. Thus grounded theory questions seek out the basic social process used to deal with a problem, phenomenology ones focus on identifying the essence of informants' experiences, and ethnographic queries explore cultural elements. Narrative questions pursue the chronology, meaning, and common experiences in participant stories, and case studies identify variables and themes within one or a few cases.

6.1.3 Replication

You may also choose to re-answer H/Qs from another study. An advantage of replication is that you can use part or all of the original study's framework, definitions, measurement tools, and methods. Replication is not only acceptable, but vital because findings from a single study are rarely conclusive. Cite the original source you are replicating.

6.2   Begin Writing Procedures

Procedures (or methods) are the step-by-step action plans for answering your H/Qs. They include a sequential explanation of when, where, and how you will conduct any intervention (described below), recruit a sample and gain subject consent (Chap. 7), and collect and analyze data (Chaps. 8 and 9). Also included is a study timeline and the time required of each participant. The more complete your details, the easier it will be for the IRB to understand your study and for you to implement it. Whether an IRB template asks for procedural information under one or many headings, give thorough details while minimizing repetition.

> **Tip.** Start Procedures with a summary sentence of design, aim, setting, and sampling, such as "This quasi-experimental, pre/post study will investigate the impact of a mindfulness class on a convenience sample of medical-surgical nurses in a 110-bed suburban hospital."

6.2.1 Describe Any Intervention

If you have no researcher-manipulated intervention, say so. If you do have one, specify who will do what, when, where, how, and how long. For example, if your intervention is postoperative gum-chewing, then state who will give exactly what type of and how much gum to what type of patients and when during the post-op trajectory, as well as how long and how many times per day each will chew gum. [Refer to the US Food & Drug Administration (FDA) website for information about testing investigational drugs and devices for FDA approval.]

6.2.2 Minimize Threats to Validity

Plan rigorous procedures to facilitate study accuracy (validity). Systematic or random threats to validity can arise from subjects, researchers, data collection, or the environment, and minimizing those threats improves study quality (Box 6.2). Report potential threats to your study when interpreting final results, and remember: No study is perfect.

Box 6.2 Minimizing Threats to Study Validity

Source	Threats (Biases)	Prevention & minimization

Subjects	• *Attrition/mortality bias*—Study dropouts share key characteristics that are then not represented in the sample
	• *Maturation bias*—Normal subject growth and development interferes with outcome measures
	• *Self-selection bias*—Self-selected samples over- or under-represent population characteristics that affect results
	• Performance biases:
	  – Individual performance errors created by transitory characteristics (e.g., tiredness or hunger)
	  – *Response set biases*—Tendency of some subjects to always agree, disagree, remain neutral, give extreme answers, or give socially acceptable answers
	  – *Hawthorne effect*—Subjects alter behavior because they are in a study
	  – Cross-contamination of groups, as when a control group starts using the intervention on their own
		• Use adequate sample size
		• Randomly select or randomize participants
		• Track number of participant refusals and withdrawals
		• Compare sample demographics to nonrespondents or population
		• Statistical analysis to remove maturation effects
		• Limit contact between study groups
		• Initial deception then debriefing of subjects
		• Placebo use

(continued)

Box 6.2 (continued)

Source	Threats (Biases)	Prevention & minimization
Researchers	• *Selection bias*—Researcher sampling creates over- or under-representation of characteristics that affect results • Inconsistent communications, timing, or context of data collection • Researchers' bias or limited self-awareness so that they affect the outcome variable	• Randomly select or randomize participants • Use consistent setting & procedures • *Blinding* researchers to experimental & control group membership • Researcher *bracketing*
Data collection/ Measurement	• Measurement bias—Inconsistent or invalid measurement of variables; poor reliability & validity of data collection tool	• Accurate (valid) & consistent (reliable) data collection tools, raters, & equipment • Calibrated equipment
Environment	• *History bias*—Major, unexpected event affecting subjects or outcome measures (e.g., pandemic or war)	• Include event as a variable or describe as context • Study replication in absence of event

6.2.3 Assess Risks, Resources, & Readiness

Finally, make sure that all your procedures are both ethical and feasible by using the three R's test of risks, resources, and readiness [1]. Ask yourself: Are participant risks reasonable or controllable, and is the risk greater to maintain the status quo or to test your intervention? Moreover, are financial, human, equipment, and time resources available, and are stakeholders ready? Too much participant risk, too few resources, or too little stakeholder buy-in can block an otherwise worthwhile study. Many researchers conduct a less than ideal project because of barriers imposed by the three R's, sometimes choosing to analyze existing data instead of collecting new data.

Next step: Choosing participants

Reference

1. Stetler CB. Updating the Stetler Model of research utilization to facilitate evidence-based practice. Nurs Outlook. 2001;49:272–9.

Plan Sample Selection & Protection 7

Key Points
- *Plan random or nonrandom sampling from your target population.*
- *The better a sample represents the population, the more generalizable are study results.*
- *All studies carry risks. Participant benefits should outweigh participant risks.*
- *Protect subjects via informed consent: Information disclosure, subject comprehension, and voluntary participation.*
- *Make sure all risks and benefits in procedures are reflected in participant consent information.*

Detail subject recruitment, selection, and protection in your protocol. The IRB's main purpose is to protect human subjects, and they judge your protocol based on written down actions, not intentions.

7.1 Select Participants

An ideal sample is the best one to answer your hypotheses/questions (H/Qs). Subjects may be people, animals, documents, equipment, events, or other. Experimental researchers often call sample members *subjects* (*Ss*), whereas others prefer the terms *respondents*, *participants*, or *informants*. Sampling is useful because we rarely can study an entire population.

© The Author(s), under exclusive license to Springer Nature Switzerland AG 2025
M. E. F. Highfield, *Doing Research*,
https://doi.org/10.1007/978-3-031-79044-7_7

Describe how you will select a sample from the larger population. A *target population* is the group to whom you want to generalize findings, while an *accessible population* is the readily available subset of that target. Your *sample* will be from the accessible population and will be more or less *representative* of the target one. The more your sample embodies all target population characteristics, the more confidently you can generalize.

When investigators do not plan to generalize study findings, ideal sampling differs. Specifically qualitative and historical researchers handpick informants who both experienced a particular phenomenon and can articulate those experiences. Such a sample is ideal for providing in-depth descriptions.

7.1.1 Random & Nonrandom Sampling

Plan either random or nonrandom sampling (Box 7.1). In *random* (*probability*) *sampling*, each member of the accessible population has an equal chance of being selected. In *nonrandom* (*non-probability*) *sampling*, some are more likely to be selected than others. For example, handpicked qualitative sampling is nonrandom.

Random selection is more cumbersome and costly, but reduces the chance of a biased sample (*selection bias*). Nonrandom selection is easier and cheaper, but yields non-generalizable findings because we must assume that subjects represent only themselves.

Adapt sampling strategies to your setting as needed. For example, randomizing a small accessible population might place everyone in the same group, and so to avoid this, start at a random point on the subject list and assign every other subject to the control or experimental group. Alternatively designate the first several recruited subjects as the control group and then assign remaining subjects to the experimental one. Unfortunately like every other element of a protocol, solving one problem creates others, so be alert to how sampling may create bias and thus, rival hypotheses. Discuss these trade-offs with your mentor now and in dissemination reports later.

Box 7.1 Random & Non-random Sampling Strategies

Types	Procedures
Probability methods	
Simple random selection	Use a random numbers table or other random method to select sample from a complete list of eligible participants.
Stratified random selection	Divide population into *strata* (groups based on age or another characteristic), then select a *proportionate or disproportionate* random sample from each stratum.
Cluster/ multistage selection	Random selection within increasingly narrow clusters. For example, randomly select US states, then cities, then households, and finally individuals by household role.
Systematic random selection	Starting at a randomly chosen point, select every nth (e.g., every 5th) individual from a complete list of potential sample members (*sampling frame*). Nth value is determined by dividing the total number on list by desired sample size.
Randomization/ random assignment	Randomly assign each eligible subject to an experimental or control group.
Non-probability methods	
Convenience/ accidental selection	Select readily available subjects. (An *inclusive convenience* sample contains all members of an accessible population.)
Snowball/ network selection	Ask each participant to identify others who meet study eligibility criteria.
Quota selection	Divide population into strata, then select a *proportionate* or *disproportionate* convenience sample from each stratum.
Purposive/ judgment selection	Handpick individuals who can describe their experiences with the phenomenon of interest. Researchers may select a *homogenous, typical, maximum variation, intense, extreme*, or *theory-based sample*.

7.1.2 Eligibility Criteria

Write out *inclusion criteria* for those who can be in your study and *exclusion criteria* for those who cannot. Common criteria relate to age, capacity, physical or psychological status, experience with a specific phenomenon, and ability to understand, speak, read, or write the primary language of the study. Narrow inclusion criteria control extraneous variables and avoid translation costs, but also create a smaller, less diverse sample. Broad criteria create opposite effects. Be able to articulate a practical, ethical, or research rationale for each eligibility criterion.

Outline specific steps in recruiting and following up with eligible participants, including how you will identify ineligible ones. Initial recruitment, for example, might be through newspapers, email, or pulling health records in a document-only study. Follow-up recruitment to improve response rate might be sending out participation reminders to the sample every few weeks during data collection. Attach verbatim copies of initial and follow-up recruitment materials as protocol appendices.

7.1.3 Sample Size

Specify your planned sample size. The ideal number is based on study design, how often the outcome variable occurs, and resource constraints like cost, time, and access to subjects. A small accessible population may be the entire sample; or a qualitative study might include less than ten handpicked informants. For a qualitative protocol specify a size range (e.g., 5–40) and explain criteria for when you will stop sampling, such as achieving data saturation or after contacting all eligible informants.

Larger samples better represent a population. In other words, the closer researchers get to sampling an entire target population, the more likely they are to capture all variations within it. Additionally large samples are needed when a study has more groups, instruments, or study variables, and when the studied variable occurs infrequently. For small studies, 30 subjects in each group may be enough to detect small to medium differences between group outcomes [1].

> **Tip.** Involve a statistician in sample size planning, or use a free online calculator like the one at https://clincalc.com/stats/samplesize.aspx. Always cite any webpage or software used.

A power analysis statistically calculates the ideal sample size for a particular experiment. It estimates a sample large enough to detect intervention effects, yet small enough to avoid wasting time and money. Power analysis calculations are based in part on the number of groups, how the outcome variable is measured, and whether researchers expect a large or small outcome difference between experimental and control groups (*effect size*).

7.2 Protect Participants

Every study creates participant risk, including subjects' stress triggered by worries about being identified with their data. Your responsibility is to identify all risks and explain how you will minimize them. Informed consent is central.

7.2.1 Informed Consent

Informed consent has three elements: Researcher disclosure of information, respondent understanding of that information, and respondent voluntary agreement to participate. Consent is a cognitive process, not an event or signed paper, and it is ongoing throughout a study. A signed form merely documents initial consent. Participants can revoke consent orally or in writing at any time without giving any reason or incurring any penalty.

> **Alert!** Consent and documentation of consent are two different things.

In procedures detail when, where, and how you will obtain consent, including any use of certified translators. Researchers must disclose Box 7.2 information in the language, vocabulary, and literacy level of participants. Attach word-for-word consent materials to the protocol, including researcher scripts for nonliterate participants.

> **Tip.** Use the Gunning Fog Index (https://www.webfx.com/tools/read-able/gunning-fog/) to identify reading level of consent documents even if reading level is generated with AI assistance.

Box 7.2 Consent Information

- Study title & investigator name(s) with affiliations
- Purpose of the study
- Selection criteria
- Study procedures
- Potential risks to subject or others
- Potential benefits to subject or others
- Subject time required
- Cost or no cost to subject
- Payments or gifts to subject or none
- Privacy protections to preserve anonymity or confidentiality
- Alternatives to participation, such as not participating or standard care
- Freedom to withdraw in part or whole without penalty
- Whether data will be kept for future studies
- How data will be secured to prevent disclosure
- The investigator's contact information to get subject questions answered
- The approving IRB's contact information for subject study concerns
- Where to get assistance if a subject feels harmed

Give eligible individuals an unthreatened opportunity to get their questions answered, to refuse participation, and to withdraw at any time. Coercion of subjects is a risk when researchers make large payments to participants or are in a position of greater power, such as supervisor-employee, teacher-student, or clinician-patient. In the protocol explain how you will minimize coercion risks through actions like maintaining subject anonymity, researcher blinding, having a neutral party obtain consent, or giving reasonable compensation.

Describe how you will document consent. Examples are a signed form, interview participation, or return of anonymous questionnaires. Your IRB may provide a standardized, customizable consent form, or you may need to write your own. (Appendix B is an editable script.) Do not collect signatures when the main study risk is identifying subjects with their data, and signatures create the only links between subjects and their data.

You may modify standard consent procedures for *minimal risk* studies or when obtaining consent would prevent doing a study. Minimal risk studies are those in which participant risk does not exceed the risks either in daily life or in routine, confidential testing. For example, IRBs may waive consent requirements for medical records studies when researchers keep data secured, de-identify records for analysis, and report only group data.

> **Tip.** If your study is minimal risk, use the IRB's minimal risk, abbreviated protocol template and consent form when available.

In rare instances when standard consent procedures would undermine research aims, an IRB may approve researchers' misleading participants (*deception*), then later *debriefing* those participants. This prevents informants from giving biased responses based on study purpose. For example, researchers studying empathy might reveal that purpose to respondents only after observing them.

Finally, use best consent practices for interview studies. Include a *process consent* option in which an interviewer may obtain mid-interview, verbal reaffirmation of consent in order to prevent the interviewee's unplanned, later-regretted sharing of illegal or sensitive information. Additionally best oral history practice is to document consent, even though such studies are typically exempt from IRB review.

7.2.2 Vulnerable Subjects

Sometimes your H/Qs are best answered by a vulnerable population. Vulnerabilities may be legal, medical, financial, social, power-inequity-related, study-related, institutional, cognitive, and communication-related [2]. CITI and OHSRP ethics training programs specify federally designated vulnerable groups who cannot legally consent, including children and patients with cognitive difficulties.

Study procedures must contain special safeguards for the rights and welfare of vulnerable subjects. For example, researchers may obtain and document both assent and consent: *Assent* (agreement) from a participant who cannot legally consent and *consent* from their legally authorized representative, parent, or guardian. In other instances when a manager is the *principal investigator* (lead researcher), that manager should be unable to discover which supervised employees participated in their study.

7.2.3 Risks & Benefits

List in the protocol any reasonably anticipated subject risks, whether physical, psychological, social, economic, legal, or other. Some IRBs ask you to estimate the likelihood, magnitude, duration, and reversibility of each, and to include risks to nonparticipants, such as family. CITI and NIH OHSRP ethics training list common risks.

Identify risks inherent in your sample recruitment, interventions, study procedures, data storage, and any sharing of data outside the institution with a statistician or during dissemination. Then, plan actions to minimize each risk, paying special attention to individual privacy and safety. State your plans to report only de-identified group data. In other situations, offer to use pseudonyms for a small, handpicked sample while informing them that they may be identifiable from their narratives. Use the term *anonymity* when even you as researcher cannot identify subjects with their data. Use the word *confidentiality* when you can connect subjects with their data but keep that information private.

> **Alert!** Collect only data to answer your H/Qs and describe key sample demographics. Never go on a curiosity-based, data "fishing expedition."

If your intervention requires participant use of a website or online application (app), then inform them that the software company may collect data and track them with "cookies" independently of your study. The app may ask user-participants to check a box that they accept tracking cookies or agree to company published policies. Disclose this information during consent, and explain how you will or will not access company-gathered data. De-identified, group data from a company can be ethically used when you are transparent with informants and the IRB.

Alert! App-collected participant data creates a privacy risk beyond your control.

Researchers must also prevent public disclosure of the 18 participant identifiers listed in the U.S. Health Insurance Portability and Accountability Act (HIPPA) as summarized in Box 7.3. HIPPA identifiers require the same privacy protections as do persons. For example, when using health record numbers to identify unique subjects secure that data in a locked device and delete those numbers before analysis.

Tip. Your institution may provide access to Research Electronic Data Capture (*REDCap*) software for secure online recruitment, distribution of questionnaires or other data collection, follow-up communications, and data analysis and storage.

Box 7.3 HIPPA Protected Information Summary [3]

- Name, including first initial/name and last name with any of the following
- Age
- Dates, except for year (e.g., birthdate, admission date)
- Contact information: Telephone, FAX, email, geographic address less than state level
- Identifier numbers or codes, such as Social Security, medical record, accounts, health plan beneficiary number, certificate/license numbers, vehicle identifiers including license plates, device identifier numbers, Internet protocol (IP) addresses
- Web URLs
- Full face photos and comparable images
- Mother's maiden name
- Biometric identifiers such as retinal scans and fingerprints

Studies create benefits, as well as risks, and subject benefits must outweigh subject risks. At a minimum respondents may benefit from knowing that their participation contributed to improved knowledge

Alert! Make sure the risks and benefits in protocol procedures match those in the consent form.

7.2.4 Subject Withdrawal

Withdrawal from intervention studies may create risk. Specify your actions to prevent harm as needed for these groups: Participants who start a study and then withdraw, those who must stop an effective intervention when the study ends, and any subjects removed from the study by investigators, such as in cases of extreme study harm. Explain any follow-up care and whether data collection from withdrawn subjects will stop or continue.

Next step: Plan data collection

References

1. Whitehead A, Julious SA, Cooper C, Campbell MJ. Estimating the sample size for a pilot randomised trial to minimise the overall trial sample size for the external pilot and main trial for a continuous outcome variable. Stat Methods Med Res. 2016;25:1057–73.
2. Gordon BG. Vulnerability in research: basic ethical concepts and general approach to review. Ochsner J. 2020;20:34–8.
3. US Department of Health & Human Services. *Protecting personal health information in research: understanding the HIPPA privacy rule*. (2003). https://privacyruleandresearch.nih.gov/pdf/HIPAA_Privacy_Rule_Booklet. pdf. Accessed 3 October 2024.

Select Data Collection Tool

8

Key Points
- *Collected data = accurate information + measurement error.*
- *Collected data are participant demographics and outcome variable measurements.*
- *Three types of data collection tools are self-reports, observational, and biophysical.*
- *The precision of quantitative tools is measured as validity and reliability.*
- *The precision of qualitative data collection using researcher-as-instrument is part of study credibility, dependability, and confirmability.*
- *Protocol procedures include the who, what, when, where, and how of data collection; instruments must be attached.*

In your protocol describe demographic and research data collection instruments, permission to use copyrighted ones, and how instruments will be distributed and collected. Full instruments and any researcher scripts must be attached as appendices.

8.1 Instrument Types

Sample demographics are usually self-reported by participants on investigator-designed forms. Questions include variables such as age, sex, ethnicity/race, education, years in clinical practice, and similar. For checklist items offer the options of "Prefer not to answer" and

"Another" with an opportunity to specify the "Another." Instructions should inform participants that they may choose not to answer any question, but that not answering may affect the usability of their data. Test any new demographic questionnaire with a few colleagues for clarity and completion time.

Three types of research instruments measure outcome variables: Self-reports, observational tools, and biophysical measures. Each has advantages and disadvantages (Box 8.1). First, self-report tools are best used to identify what people think and feel, and examples are questionnaires, interviews, focus groups, and diaries. Self-report questions may be (1) closed-ended with fixed response options, such as multiple choice questions, (2) semi-structured, such as fill-in-the blank questions or interview topic guides, or (3) open-ended in order to let respondents determine the direction of their answers, such as "Tell me about [X]." Second, observational tools are useful in gathering data about behaviors, conditions, and events. Examples include narrative field notes or checklists with items that are mutually exclusive (not overlapping) and collectively exhaustive (covering all possible options). Third, biophysical tools like monitors, lab equipment, and fitness trackers yield objective, equipment-mediated data.

Box 8.1 Data Collection Tools: Advantages & Disadvantages

	Self-reports	Observational	Biophysical
Advantages	Questionnaires cost less money, time, & effort than interviews. Compared to questionnaires interviews avoid literacy issues, allow observation, have higher response rates, & are more flexible. Focus group members may facilitate each other.	Direct observation of some variables is more accurate than self-reports. Participant observers (data collectors) who are members of the observed group gain insider (*emic*) perspectives. Non-participant observers gain outsider (*etic*) perspectives.	Minimize researcher or response set bias.

(continued)

Box 8.1 (continued)

	Self-reports	Observational	Biophysical
Disad-vantages	Written questionnaires limit follow-up. Longer questionnaires yield lower response rates. Interviews require expensive recording equipment & transcription.* Interviewer bias or informant response set biases may interfere. Focus group members may inhibit each other.	Participant observers may lose objectivity, & non-participant ones may not fully understand their observations. Observer training & establishing observer intra- & inter-rater reliability (consistency) may be costly. Subjects who are aware of being observed may exhibit the Hawthorne effect.	Equipment & its calibration, user training, & establishing inter-equipment reliability (consistency) may be costly. Data recorded by subjects may be biased.

*Transcripts generated by online meeting software and new electronic transcription services reduce costs

If your study's conceptual framework has a complementary data collection instrument, use it. Otherwise search for a relevant tool in published instrument books or online professional databases. Ask for librarian assistance or search using "[name of your outcome variable] AND research instruments." Alternatively use the *CINAHL* database pull-down "publication type" menu for "research instrument" and "questionnaire/scale."

Obtain author permission to use any instrument. Some copyrighted tools are available only with author consent and for a fee, while many are free to those conducting academic or noncommercial studies. Some instruments are free to anyone. Tool authors may ask you only to submit your collected raw (unanalyzed) data to them, a reasonable request that allows them to continue examining the instrument's reliability and validity.

If no instrument measures your outcome variable(s), consult your mentor. Options are to modify an existing tool with author permission, study different variables, or conduct methodological research to develop a new valid and reliable instrument.

Alert! You can research only what you can measure.

8.2   Examine Tool Precision

The best tools measure study variables directly, accurately, and consistently. A direct instrument measures the variable itself, while an indirect tool measures the variable obliquely through something else. Moreover, a direct measure of one variable may be an indirect measure of another. To illustrate, weight is measured directly by a scale and indirectly by self-report, while adult pain is measured directly by self-report and indirectly by observing behaviors. Instruments must also consistently measure the right variable.

Alert! Collected data = accurate information + measurement error

8.2.1 Quantitative Tools

The best quantitative instruments demonstrate strong statistical validity and reliability. *Validity* is a tool's accuracy in measuring a variable (Box 8.2), while *reliability* is its consistency (Box 8.3). Validity is like hitting the bull's-eye on a target, and reliability is consistently hitting that bull's-eye. Reliability and validity are measured on a continuum, and the higher they are, the better your data will be. Direct measures are more likely to be valid and reliable because they reduce effects of *mediating*, *moderating*, and extraneous variables.

Box 8.2 Tool Validity

Validity	Description	Procedures	Statistics
Face validity	**Expert opinion** of tool accuracy	Tool items look valid to experts	N/A
Content validity	**Comprehensiveness** of tool: Do items include all possible items measuring the variable?	Researchers identify all possible items from literature. An expert panel scores how well each item matches the variable's conceptual definition	Items accepted based on majority agreement of experts. Alternatively item & scale content validity indices (CVI) are calculated with acceptable CVI ≥ 0.78
Construct validity	**Conceptual accuracy** of tool as: **1) Factor analysis:** What dimensions of the variable are represented by items?	Similar items are grouped together statistically, then researchers label each group (factor)	Factor analysis
	2) Convergent validity: Is there a relationship between scores of tools measuring the same thing?	Ss complete two different tools measuring the same variable (e.g., two different joyful scales)	Positive correlation of $r \geq 0.50^*$
	3) Discriminant validity: Are scores of tools measuring dissimilar concepts unrelated?	All Ss complete tools measuring dissimilar variables (e.g., joyful & depression scales)	No or low correlation $(r)^\dagger$
	4) Known groups validity: Does the tool discriminate between those who demonstrate the variable & those who do not?	A group demonstrating the variable (e.g., joy) & one not demonstrating it (e.g., depressed) complete the same joyful tool	Inverse $(-)$, no (0), or low correlation (r); or ANOVA or t-test scores differ

(continued)

Box 8.2 (continued)

Validity	Description	Procedures	Statistics
Criterion validity	**Relationship of tool to criteria:** **1) Predictive** validity: Do tool scores accurately predict a future criterion? **2) Concurrent** validity: Are tool scores related to a coexisting or gold standard criterion?	Tool scores compared to 1) Future valid criterion (e.g., does GRE predict graduate school grades) 2) Present valid criterion (e.g., are new pain tool scores related to pain self-report)	Strong correlation with r closer to +1.0 or to −1.0

[*]r values reflect both direction & strength of variables' relationship. Strength is closeness to an absolute value of 1.0, & direction is (+) or (−). For example, $r = -0.92$ indicates a strong, inverse/negative relationship
[†]No correlation is $r = 0$. Low correlations are closer to $r = 0$

Box 8.3 Tool Reliability

Reliability	Description	Statistical tests	Desired values
Internal consistency	**Item** consistency: Do all items measure the same concept/variable?	Cronbach's α (alpha); or Split-half correlation (r)	α or $r \geq$ 0.70 acceptable α or $r \geq$ 0.80 good α or $r \geq$ 0.90 strong[†]

(continued)

Box 8.3 (continued)

Reliability	Description	Statistical tests	Desired values
Interrater & intra-rater reliability	**Data collector** consistency: Are multiple rater scores similar? Are scores of the same rater consistent?	Correlation (r) between rater scores; percent agreement; or Cohen's kappa (κ)[¶]	$r \geq 0.41$ moderate $r \geq 0.61$ substantial $r \geq 0.81$ near perfect. Or $\kappa \leq 0$ no agreement $\kappa \geq 0.61$ substantial agreement
Stability	**Time** consistency: Does the tool measure consistently over time?	Correlation (r) between test & retest scores	$r \geq 0.40$ fair $r \geq 0.60$ good $r \geq 0.75$ excellent
Parallel forms	**Version** consistency: Are scores on different forms/versions of the same tool similar?	Correlation (r) between different forms of the tool	$r \geq 0.70$ acceptable $r \geq 0.80$ good $r \geq 0.90$ strong

[†]Perfect internal consistency Cronbach's $\alpha = 1.0$; no internal consistency Cronbach's $\alpha = 0$; α or $r \geq 0.95$ indicates possible redundant items
[¶]$\kappa = 1.0$ if perfect agreement

Reliability and validity are in a tool's manual, methodological studies, and the methods sections of research reports. In your protocol cite primary sources, and include type and values of reliability and validity, such as "Cronbach $\alpha = .91$." For extensively tested tools, like the GRE or MMPI, note that "reliability and validity are well-established."

Also name the population in which reliability and validity were established, such as students or oncology patients. You can use the tool with other groups, but be transparent about this. Either way, plan to run tool reliability statistics on your own study data.

Alert! A tool may be useful even if not ideal. Financial, time, and equipment resources affect tool selection.

8.2.2 Qualitative Tools & More

The accuracy of a qualitative instrument is judged in the context of the study's dependability, confirmability, and credibility (earlier Box 5.4). Statistical validity and reliability do not apply. The researcher-as-instrument often modifies a qualitative topic guide or questionnaire during interviews in order to follow up on participant leads. Thus, qualitative instruments are flexible, responsive, and not locked into predetermined questions. Finally, instruments used in methodological research and mixed methods are judged by relevant quantitative or qualitative criteria, and assessing quality historical data collection is described elsewhere [1].

8.3   A Few Practical Matters

For best response rate, make respondent participation as quick and easy as possible. Develop data collection procedures that anticipate how sample characteristics might affect response rate. For example, online questionnaires accessed by scanning a QR code work well for a computer savvy population, but others may prefer a mailed copy with a researcher self-addressed, stamped envelope for return. Additionally, put written materials in this priority order: Consent information, research questionnaire, and then demographic question-naire. If conducting interviews or collecting biophysical data, then make the process as convenient and comfortable as possible. Always give accurate estimates of time required. Finally, make fol-low-up communications inviting, thank respondents, and if funded give participants some form of noncoercive gift or compensation.

Next step: Plan data analysis

Reference

1. Lewenson SB, Herrmann EK, editors. Capturing nursing history: a guide to historical methods in research. New York: Springer; 2008.

Propose Data Analysis

9

Key Points
- *Quantitative data are analyzed using descriptive and inferential statistics.*
- *An appropriate statistical test is chosen based on the hypothesis/ question (H/Q), sampling, and type of data.*
- *Qualitative data are analyzed by researchers' immersion in data and critical reflection.*

The three purposes of data analysis are to describe sample demographics, to describe variables, and to answer your H/Qs. Quantitative analysis is rigid, statistical, and conducted after a set of data are collected, while qualitative analysis is flexible, requires critical reflection, and may begin during data collection.

> **Tip**. To increase your confidence, focus on mastering only the specific statistical or qualitative analysis needed for your project. Begin by completing the "Data Analysis" section of the Protocol Worksheet.

For the IRB it may be enough to write a general statement that you will use descriptive and/or inferential statistics or to name a qualitative analysis strategy dictated by study design. For your own use, however, you should identify specific statistical tests or qualitative analytic steps now. This chapter guides you through the basics of quantitative then qualitative analysis.

9.1 Quantitative Analysis

Quantitative data are divided into four types: Nominal, ordinal, interval, and ratio (Box 9.1). Nominal data are categories that can only be counted; they are the least analyzable type. Ordinal, then interval, then ratio data permit increasingly more precise analyses. For that reason interval or ratio data are preferred. Nonetheless, some variables can be measured only nominally or ordinally.

Box 9.1 Data Levels: From Low to High

Level	Example	Characteristics
1. *Nominal data*—Categories without any mathematical or ranked value	Country of origin	*Discrete data* that occur only in categories or whole numbers[*]
2. *Ordinal data*—Data that can be placed in a meaningful order, but without equal intervals between values	0–10 pain scale	
3. *Interval data*—Data that can be placed in a meaningful order with equal intervals between values, but no absolute zero	Fahrenheit temperature scale	*Continuous data* that have decimal point or fractional values
4. *Ratio data*—Data that can be placed in a meaningful order with equal intervals between values and an absolute zero	Hours worked per day	

[*]Ordinal data are sometimes analyzed as continuous data, as for example, when ordinal pain scores are averaged and reported as fractional values (e.g., 5.7)

Tip. Include data level when describing your instrument, for example, "SWBS is an ordinal scale." Find this information in the tool manual or methodological studies.

Some label qualitative data as nominal. Quantitative analysis of nominal data, however, requires counting frequencies, such as how many subjects have blue or brown eyes. In contrast qualitative analysis requires in-depth descriptions, without numbers.

If possible include a statistician during study planning. If you wait until after data collection, you risk the unpleasant discovery that you should have collected data differently. Statisticians suggest relevant statistical tests, ways to collect higher level data, and how to record *raw data* for analysis—usually a spreadsheet with individual subjects on rows and data questions in columns. (See Protocol Worksheet.) Confer with the statistician about their role in analyzing data and writing results. The following information will help you communicate with a statistician or plan your own analysis. Student researchers may be expected to analyze their own data.

> **<u>Tip.</u>** If your facility has no consulting statistician, ask your mentor or local university about *gratis* or paid statistical support.

9.1.1 Descriptive vs. Inferential Statistics

Quantitative data are analyzed using descriptive (Box 9.2) and inferential statistics. *Descriptive statistics* describe one variable at a time (*univariate analysis*) or the associations between two or more variables (*bivariate* or *multivariate analyses*). In contrast, *inferential statistics* allow researchers to draw inferences by testing hypotheses.

Box 9.2 Common Descriptive Tests

Statistic (Population & sample symbols)[*]	Description
Frequency of data	
Frequency (N, n)	How often a variable occurs (e.g., 4 times or $n = 4$)
Percent (%)	Frequency translated into percentage (e.g., 4 persons divided by sample total of 89 = 4.5%)
How data cluster together (*central tendency of data*)	
Mean (μ, $\bar{x}$ or M)	Average number or score

(continued)

Box 9.2 (continued)

Statistic (Population & sample symbols)*	Description
Median (η, x or Mdn)	Middle number when scores are rank ordered; if there are 2 middle numbers, the median is the average of those 2
Mode (M_o)	Most frequently occurring number or score
How data spread out (*data distribution*)	
Range (R)	High score minus low score
Standard deviation (σ; *SD*)	How far data vary from the mean score; includes positive and negative distance from the mean
Standard error (SE)	How much the sample mean differs from the population mean
Bivariate or multivariate associations	
Correlations (*r*)	Shows the relationships between 2 or more variables

*Use sample symbols in your project report. Exception is N = entire sample and n = subset

Descriptive statistics may also be displayed as graphs. Common frequency graphs are pie charts and bar graphs, while clustering and distribution of data may be depicted in a line or bar graph. Scatterplots show the relationship between at least two variables. Line graphs may show a normal bell curve, a peaked bell curve with a narrow range, a flattened bell curve with wide range, or a skewed curve with data bunching up on one end and a long "arm" of data stretching out either to right (right skewed) or to the left (left skewed).

An inferential test is selected based on four criteria: Whether an H/Q is simple or complex, the outcome variable's level of data, the number of subject groups, and whether those groups contain the same persons (*paired* or *dependent groups*) or different persons (*unpaired* or *independent groups*). Moreover, inferential tests are divided into parametric and nonparametric tests (Box 9.3). *Parametric statistics* require higher interval or ratio data from adequately sized, randomly selected samples that represent a larger population. *Nonparametric statistics* may be used with any level of data when the sample is small and nonrandom.

Box 9.3 Common Inferential Tests

Parametric	Nonparametric alternatives
Correlation tests for relationships [*]	
Pearson's r (*r*)—tests strength & direction of a relationship between 2 variables	Spearman's rho (*r*)—tests strength & direction of a relationship between 2 variables
Experimental tests for differences	
Independent/unpaired *t*-test (*t*)—tests for differences between the *means* of 2 groups with different subjects (Ss)	Mann-Whitney U (*U*)—tests for differences between *medians* of 2 groups with different Ss (ordinal data)
Dependent/paired *t*-test (*t*)— tests for differences between *means* of 2 groups with the same Ss (e.g., pretest/posttest)	Wilcoxon signed rank (Z)—tests for differences between *medians* of 2 groups with the same Ss (ordinal data)
Analysis of variance or ANOVA (*F*)—tests for differences between means of ≥ 3 independent groups of different Ss	Kruskal-Wallis (*H*)—Tests for differences between *medians* of ≥ 3 independent groups of different Ss (ordinal data)
	Chi-square statistic (χ^2)—tests for differences in *frequencies* between ≥ 2 independent groups of different Ss (nominal data)

[*]*r* (relationship) strength is its closeness to 1.0; direction is (+) or (−)

9.1.2 Significance Level

When testing a hypothesis, select a *p* value (significance level). That *p* is your benchmark for determining whether or not the statistically calculated results *p* supports your hypothesis or correlation. Common researcher-set *p* values are $p \leq 0.01$ and $p \leq 0.05$. The symbol "≤" means less than or equal to. In contrast, statistical results *p* values are reported as exact numbers using the "=" symbol (e.g., $p = 0.021$). If the calculated results *p* is less than or equal to your preset *p*, then you can accept the hypothesis or correlation as true. Otherwise reject it as false.

Choose your preset *p* value based on study risks. A common $p \leq 0.05$ means a willingness to accept the odds that 5 times out of 100, study results are wrong. In experiments with high risk interventions, investigators are more rigorous, presetting a lower $p \leq 0.01$. This means they are willing to be wrong only 1 time out of 100. A $p \leq 0.01$ makes them unlikely to accept a false hypothesis, a mistake that could lead to dangerous, non-beneficial treatment. In exploratory very low risk studies, however, researchers sometimes preset a high $p \leq 0.10$ in order to err on the side of accepting a wrong hypothesis; the benefit is stimulating more research.

Here's an example. When a preset $p \leq 0.05$ is compared to a statistical result of $p = 0.02$, researchers accept the hypothesis. But when a more rigorous preset $p \leq 0.01$ is compared to the same calculated $p = 0.02$, researchers reject the hypothesis.

9.1.2.1 Data Safety and Monitoring Plan (DSMP)

A DSMP (data safety and monitoring plan) is required for high risk, intervention protocols. It is not applicable to surveys, low risk experiments, or qualitative studies. A DSMP includes responsibilities of research team members in monitoring, reporting, and investigating serious adverse events.

> **Tip.** Templates and guidance for DSMPs are available through nih.gov and hhs.gov websites and from research institutions.

9.2   Qualitative Analysis

Qualitative data analysis requires researcher immersion in the data to uncover its meaning based on study design (Box 9.4). Also, instead of collaborating with statisticians, qualitative researchers join forces with colleagues or informants. Accurate results are facilitated by contrasting and comparing multiple data sources (*data triangulation*), independent then combined analysis by multiple researchers (*researcher triangulation*), and finally verifying results with participants (*member checks*).

Box 9.4 Qualitative Analyses

Design	Data examples	Analysis [1]
Case study or case series	Texts, Images, Interviews, Observations	In-depth description of one to four cases (persons, events, or phenomena) within boundaries of a particular time & place.
Ethnography	Observation, Recordings, Images, Artifacts, Field notes, Maps	Describe actors, characteristics, & processes of a culture or subculture. Draw or photograph setting. Identify recurrent themes & patterns. Generate new theory or compare data to existing theory. May involve concurrent data collection & analysis (*constant comparison*).
Grounded Theory	Interviews with 20–30 informants	Coding data with constant comparison until data saturation. Common analytic methods: Glaser & Strauss (classic), Strauss & Corbin, & Charmaz.
Narrative	Stories, diaries, images from one or more informants	Thematic, structural, contextual, or visual analysis to uncover chronology, key events, & larger meaning of the story. Sometimes writing informants' stories into one chronology.
Phenomen-ology	Interviews with 5–25+ informants	Researcher brackets, reads & re-reads data, & uncovers themes related to informant experiences of what happened & how. Synthesizes themes into one statement of the "essence" of experiences. Common analytic methods: Colaizzi, Giorgi, or Van Kaam.
[Unidentified qualitative design] †	Interviews, written or oral narratives with a few informants	Immersion in data to identify emerging & recurrent themes or concepts & their relationships related to study purpose (*content analysis*). Sometimes researcher or data triangulation.

†Weaker investigations outside the five major qualitative traditions

Next steps: Gain approval and start the study!

Reference

1. Creswell JW, Poth C. Qualitative inquiry and research design: choosing among five approaches. 4th ed. Los Angeles: Sage; 2018.

Conduct the Study

10

Key Points

- *Submit your completed research protocol to the IRB.*
- *After receiving written IRB approval, begin the study.*
- *Obtain additional IRB authorization before making any mid-study changes to the protocol.*
- *After beginning your IRB-approved study, you may need to overcome challenges of limited time, flagging motivation, your own inadvertent mistakes, and unexpected concurrent events.*

10.1 Get IRB Approval

A well-written protocol will both gain swift IRB approval and give you step-by-step procedures for conducting your study. Before submitting to the IRB, format references consistently, check spelling, and ask your mentor for final critique.

If planning a pilot study as a small-scale, methodological test of your research procedures before your full study, submit a pilot research protocol to the IRB for their approval. Then after you learn from the pilot, you can submit the new and improved full study protocol. Alternatively, you may include the pilot as step one and the full study protocol as step two of a single IRB application. However, this may be less efficient because any change to the full protocol after IRB approval requires additional IRB authorization.

© The Author(s), under exclusive license to Springer Nature Switzerland AG 2025
M. E. F. Highfield, *Doing Research*,
https://doi.org/10.1007/978-3-031-79044-7_10

If you are a student, provide the research-site IRB with a copy of the university IRB approval letter. When doing multisite research, one IRB will be designated as primary; seek its approval first and then submit that approved protocol to all sites. Should a secondary data collection site request protocol changes, the primary site must approve those modifications. Consult your mentor or primary IRB for questions.

Each IRB assigns a number to your protocol and then approves it or requests changes. Read IRB communications carefully, follow directions exactly, and keep copies of all correspondence. Once approved, begin your study.

Alert! You as the principal investigator are ultimately responsible for the legal and ethical conduct of your study. IRBs approve a written plan, but you are responsible for enacting it.

10.2 Meet the Challenges

Conducting a study has its challenges. Presumably you already balanced ideal study procedures with actual risks, resources, and stakeholder readiness [1]. Still, things may go wrong. In a dramatic example, the COVID-19 pandemic created new contingencies not only for care, but also for in-progress research.

If the unexpected happens address it immediately. In consultation with your mentor, halt the study if necessary, and report the issue and proposed solutions to the IRB. Include any new risks to subjects, such as a privacy breach, or threats to *data integrity*. An example of a data integrity threat is broadening sample inclusion criteria after starting data collection. In that case you changed your approved protocol and data are from two different samples, so be transparent with mentor, IRB, and statistician, as well as in dissemination reports. If the issue and its solution create no foreseeable subject risks or data integrity threats, notify all approving IRBs anyway. When in doubt, consult!

Alert! Report unanticipated negative participant effects to the IRB as soon as you become aware. If needed request protocol modifications.

Time is also a challenge for clinician-researchers whose primary role is patient care. Hours spent writing a protocol can be flexed around a work schedule, but enacting the study requires being available when potential subjects are. Consider adjusting your time expectations for study completion. You may also add a research team member by submitting an IRB protocol modification that identifies the person's study role and proof of ethics training.

Alert! Keep a count of potential subjects missed. Record on your data sheet those who consented but withdrew or were lost to follow-up. (See Protocol Worksheet.) Report these numbers during dissemination because they create attrition or selection biases.

Another barrier is flagging motivation. Perhaps you spent so much energy on planning that you are tired of looking at your study. To overcome this, set a 10 minute timer and take only the next procedural step. You can't do a study all at once anyway, so don't take on that psychological burden.

Mistakes also happen. Researchers may absent-mindedly violate their own protocols. If this happens to you, the way to make it worse is to avoid facing your errors. The way to make it better is to communicate promptly with your mentor and the IRB about the mistake, a proposed solution, and any new subject or data integrity risks. Follow IRB feedback. Never cover up mistakes, or you may be accused of intentional misconduct. Make things right. Be transparent.

Tip. Keep dated, written records of any study changes for dissemination reports.

Next step: Time for answers

Reference

1. Stetler CB. Updating the Stetler Model of research utilization to facilitate evidence-based practice. Nurs Outlook. 2001;49:272–9.

Analyze Data & Interpret Results

11

Key Points
- *Clean quantitative data, and analyze them with appropriate descriptive and inferential statistics.*
- *Interpret statistical results to answer each hypothesis or research question (H/Q).*
- *Reporting results and interpreting results are two separate steps in quantitative studies; they are more integrated in qualitative ones.*
- *Analyze qualitative data by reflective immersion in order to identify emerging ideas that match study purpose.*

Finally it's time to answer your H/Qs! Take this in three stages. First, describe demographic and any quantitative outcome variables one at a time, and calculate participant response rate. Second, analyze study variables related to each H/Q (i.e., results), and finally, answer each H/Q by interpreting what those results mean.

11.1 Quantitative Methods

11.1.1 Preparation

First, if working with a statistician, confirm that you both understand how raw data are recorded. Then one of you will clean data. Cleaning includes dealing with missing data, assuring consistent variable labels, deleting duplicate data, and managing extreme data (*outliers*). Some

© The Author(s), under exclusive license to Springer Nature Switzerland AG 2025
M. E. F. Highfield, *Doing Research*,
https://doi.org/10.1007/978-3-031-79044-7_11

software automatically compensates for missing data, or you can fill in blanks with the average score of other respondents. If any subject omitted too many answers, that row on the spreadsheet may be omitted from analysis; count any omissions. Next, make sure that all data for each variable are listed under the exact same variable name, and finally, identify any participants with extreme outlier data so that analysis can be adjusted as below.

11.1.2 Analysis

Calculate the response rate as the percentage of subjects who participated from the total sample. Then use descriptive statistics (earlier Box 9.2) to summarize each demographic and outcome variable and to answer descriptive research questions. Follow this with inferential analyses (earlier Box 9.3) to test correlations or hypotheses. Compare each inferentially calculated p value to your preset p, and if it is less than the preset p, accept your correlation or hypothesis as true; results are statistically significant. Otherwise reject it; results are likely due to chance.

> **Tip.** Although rejecting a hypothesis or correlation feels disappointing, it can lead to new research questions. Remember that you are seeking knowledge, not proof of preconceptions.

Calculate inferential results both with and without outliers. If the outliers create excessive distortion in results, omit those subjects as atypical, and note those deletions in final reports. Otherwise leave them in for a larger, more diverse sample. Another option is to report results both with and without outliers when those results differ. A statistician can help make these judgments.

> **Tip.** If you collected data using REDCap software, use REDCap for descriptive analyses and then export data to Excel or SPSS software for inferential testing. Protect data privacy as approved by the IRB.

RESULTS FROM SAMPLE

		Statistically significant relationship (results $p \leq$ preset p)	*No statistically significant relationship* (results $p \geq$ preset p)
REALITY IN POPULATION	*Relationship exists between variables*	Accurate results	False negative results (<u>Type II error</u>)
	No relationship between variables	False positive results (<u>Type I error</u>)	Accurate results

Fig. 11.1 Statistical validity

11.1.3 Interpreting Results

Interpret statistical results to answer each H/Q. Ideally research results reflect reality, and perhaps that will be true for your study. Nonetheless, research cannot prove something beyond doubt, so consider these four issues when interpreting quantitative results: Statistical validity (calculated results reflect reality), clinical meaningfulness of findings (*clinical significance*), internal validity (confidence in answers to hypotheses), and external validity (generalizability).

Statistical validity is your confidence that statistical results accurately reflect reality. Unfortunately p values are not foolproof, and you cannot know whether your results include Type I or II errors (Fig. 11.1). A clinical analogy for these errors is that a Type I error is like a false positive COVID-19 test that shows a healthy person is infected, while a Type II error is like a false negative COVID-19 test that shows no disease in an infected person. Always discuss your study results in tentative terms.

Tip. Statisticians describe a Type I error as rejecting a true null hypothesis, and a Type II error as accepting a false null hypothesis.

Clinical meaningfulness of results is when the intervention created important, "genuine, palpable effects" for individuals, groups, or healthcare decisions whether or not results were statistically significant. [1, p. 449] Researchers sometimes plan quantifiable measures of clinical significance into their studies.

Tip. Researchers focus on populations, while treating clinicians often focus on individuals. Thus, clinical meaningfulness is relevant to clinicians using research results.

Individual clinical meaningfulness consists of one of these: Meeting improvement benchmarks set by experts, patient-perceived improvements, or care improvements that don't add problems [1]. Data outliers, anecdotal observations, or qualitative data may provide evidence.

Group clinical meaningfulness includes statistical estimates of one of these three: Average group benefit, a range of outcomes within which benefits may occur (*confidence interval*), or the *number needed to treat* (NNT) [1]. NNT is how many patients must receive an intervention over a set time in order to help one additional person.

Alert! Clinically meaningful results may not be statistically significant, and statistically significant results may not be clinically meaningful.

Internal and external validity reflect study rigor. Internal validity is how much confidence you have in the finding of a statistical cause-and-effect relationship between hypothesis variables, and external validity is generalizability of results (earlier Box 5.3). When considering these, decide how well your procedures controlled extraneous variables and minimized threats to validity (earlier Box 6.2).

11.2   Qualitative Methods

Each qualitative design prescribes unique data preparation, analysis, and interpretation (earlier Box 9.4). Generally, however, data preparation involves organizing data files, such as sorting interview transcripts by type or chronology. Then integrated analysis and interpretation require researchers' immersion in data in order to uncover emerging themes. When reading data, researchers underline key sentences and jot memos and codes in the margins. Memos add ideas and references, while codes group data into categories that can be combined into fewer themes. Investigators seek to avoid their own and subject response set biases during this process. They also may value equally the ideas raised by one or many informants because qualitative projects focus on the breadth and depth of a phenomenon, not on counting frequencies.

> **Tip.** Qualitative analysis software organizes data, but researchers must analyze and interpret their meaning. At present artificial intelligence software, like free Perplexity (https://www.perplexity.ai/), support but cannot yet replace human analysis.

11.3 Adapted Quantitative & Qualitative Methods

Mixed methods, methodological, ideological, and historical researchers adapt quantitative and qualitative analytic methods to their purposes. Mixed methods and methodological researchers use both quantitative and qualitative analyses as described above, but in mixed methods complementary quantitative and qualitative results inform each other within a single study (earlier Box 3.3) and yield integrated interpretations that answer H/Qs. In contrast, ideological investigators operate within an advocacy paradigm and so analyze both quantitative and qualitative data from within specific ways of thinking, such as gender theory. They may also involve respondents in analyzing their own data, as in participatory action research. Different from these groups are historians who answer questions using descriptive, analytic, interpretive, or comparative methods to examine primary and secondary source data within the data's historical context [2], rather than within the researcher's contemporary context (*presentism*).

Next step: Share your findings

References

1. Polit DF, Beck CT. Nursing research: generating and assessing evidence for nursing practice. 10th ed. Philadelphia: Wolters Kluwer; 2017.
2. Lewenson SB, Herrmann EK, editors. Capturing nursing history: a guide to historical methods in research. New York: Springer; 2008.

Disseminate Findings!

12

Key Points
- *The research process isn't complete until you share findings.*
- *Close out your study with the IRB, other approving bodies, grantors, or individuals.*
- *Write an abstract using relevant protocol content; add results, discussion, and conclusion.*
- *Follow author guidelines for posters, presentations, and publications.*
- *Beware of predatory conferences and journals.*

Telling others about your research outcomes is cause for celebration. Not only may results improve patient and provider lives, but they also promote further study. Make it a priority to share findings at the research site. Then disseminate your work to wider local, national, or international audiences, including lay ones. You want your findings to be used, your study replicated, and your informants to feel valued—you wouldn't have a study without them!

12.1 Close Your Study

Begin dissemination by closing out your study with the IRB, other approving bodies, and grantors. Notify the IRB and other groups about project completion, accompanied by an abstract. The abstract should include a clear statement of the problem and its significance, study purpose, hypotheses/research questions (H/Qs), procedures, results, discussion, implications, and conclusion. Additionally, send a cover letter and abstract to subjects if promised. After closure disseminate findings through conferences and publications targeting your university, healthcare system, and relevant professional and lay organizations.

12.2 Present at a Conference

Tip. It takes no more time to prepare in advance than at the last minute.

Conference posters and presentations require submitting an abstract for competitive peer-review and usually membership in the sponsoring organization. Organizers may accept only previously unpublished studies. Expect to rewrite your existing abstract to conform exactly to conference instructions for headings, structure, word count, and deadlines. If you do not, your work will be rejected. Ask your mentor to critique your abstract, and submit it well before the deadline to avoid software glitches.

Tip. Editing assistance is available through libraries with Grammarly or similar software, free AI if allowable, and at fee-for-service websites.

12.2.1 Posters

If your abstract is accepted for a poster, meticulously follow display instructions related to font size, poster size, display requirements (e.g., tabletop space or hanging), and so on. Then during conference poster sessions, stand nearby to engage viewers.

Posters are visual media and should communicate your entire project at a glance. They are not articles pasted on posterboard. Your poster should attract attention, stimulate networking, and have easy to follow main points. Make clear the problem you wanted to solve, what you found, and study implications. Use a statement, picture, or graph as a focal point for your main message, as in the "Got Milk?"

U.S. dairy campaign. A well-done poster should stand alone without you (Box 12.1).

Box 12.1 Poster Tips & Tricks

- Free online PowerPoint® templates facilitate poster creation in the required size.
- Copy centers can create either foam board or travel-friendly roll-up posters from your PowerPoint® pdf.
- Use your organization's required logo, colors, & formatting.
- Follow required or research process headings.
- Make the title readable from 4 feet. Consider font of ~36 point for headings & ~24 point for text. Keep font style & size consistent.
- Include author names with contact information for a corresponding author.
- Use bullet points, active voice, phrases (not sentences), pictures, & two-dimensional, color-blind-friendly graphs.
- Use white (negative) space to highlight key points.
- Use color to direct the viewer stepwise through poster content or to highlight key points.
- Avoid jargon, define acronyms, check spelling & grammar, & remove the irrelevant & redundant.
- Use a free QR code-generating website to add a code for supplemental information, like abstract or a poster pdf on *digital commons*.
- Make your business cards available near the poster.

Tip. To refine your poster draft, score it yourself using online criteria like Harvard's "Rubric for Scientific Posters" (https://writingcenter.catalyst.harvard.edu/files/catalystwcc/files/rubric_for_scientific_posters_harvard_catalyst.pdf).

12.2.2 Podium Presentations

After abstract acceptance follow conference instructions about content, available audiovisual equipment, presentation length, and deadlines. Expect to submit slides a week or more in advance. Prepare early, invite mentor critique, and practice, practice, practice. If part of a panel confer with the moderator. Make sure you are clear on technical requirements of the venue and presentation software.

Visual media like PowerPoint® slides can highlight key points. Use phrases, adequate font size, and bullet points. Avoid tiny print, unreadable graphs, or distracting animation. Detailed descriptions are best in your spoken words or a handout.

> **Tip.** Always be prepared to present without your slides in case they don't work.

Before your session make sure that your slides load properly. If you brought an updated version on a flash drive, include your name in the file label. Load the file onto the presentation computer desktop for easy access, and then test it.

During the presentation use *printed* PowerPoint® "Notes" view that shows your slide at the top and speaker content below. Alternatively set up the presentation computer so you, but not the audience, can see the "Notes" view electronically. Practicing in advance will keep you within your assigned time. Avoid the temptation to ad lib, and always leave a few minutes for questions. If you finish early and no one has questions, ask the audience how they might use your findings.

> **Alert!** Never exceed your allotted presentation time. Going over disrespects other presenters and precludes fruitful discussion.

12.2.3 Predatory Conferences

Sadly not all conferences are created equal. Some are predatory and their organizers seek to profit from your time, money, and energy without benefiting you. Disseminating through legitimate conferences or publications often triggers an onslaught of emails from probable predatory conferences, such as the "World Congress" of this and that. Investigate before investing effort.

> **Tip.** See the University of Wisconsin Ebling Library's online "Where Should I Publish? : Identifying Predatory Conferences" (https://researchguides.library.wisc.edu/c.php?g=1154500&p=8431828).

12.3 Write for Publication

12.3.1 Find a Journal

Publication in a peer-reviewed journal facilitates widest dissemination. Some researchers pursue publication in journals reporting a high (10) or good (3) impact factor on a 0–10 scale that measures how frequently the journal is cited. For beginning clinical researchers, however, impact factors are nice but unnecessary because databases like PubMed and CINAHL make peer-reviewed articles available to anyone. Pick a journal whose purpose and readership fits your project (Box 12.2). Some journals focus on clinical practice, others on education or administration, and still others on research; adapt writing of your research project to the relevant journal audience.

Box 12.2 Find a Journal

- Copy & paste your abstract into Journal/Author Name Estimator (JANE) (https://jane.biosemantics.org/) to retrieve relevant, PubMed-listed journals.
- Search the Directory of Open Access Journals (DOAJ) (https://doaj.org).
- Check your protocol references for relevant journals.
- Identify relevant specialty organization journal(s).
- Search discipline-related publisher lists (e.g., Wiley's *Directory of Nursing Journals.*)

12.3.2 Predatory Journals

Like conferences not all journals are created equal. In particular open access ones may be legitimate or predatory. Predatory ones charge author fees, have poor quality peer-review if any, are not listed in credible databases like PubMed and CINAHL, and may remove work from their online sites without warning. Never sign over copyright of your article to a suspected predatory journal.

> **Tip.** A volunteer developed, current list of predatory publishers and predatory journals is at https://predatoryjournals.org/the-list.

Fortunately the independent, nonprofit DOAJ [1] identifies quality, open-access, peer-reviewed journals and grants its seal of approval to those meeting seven quality criteria. If you find an open access journal that shows the DOAJ symbol but is not listed in DOAJ, then send that information to DOAJ as your contribution toward maintaining scientific rigor.

12.3.3 Write Well

After selecting a peer-reviewed journal, conform your article exactly to its author instructions about headings, formatting, and submission. Within the selected journal, find one or two research reports that used the same design that you used, and print them as models.

> **Alert!** Submit your manuscript to only one journal at a time.

To begin a draft, copy and paste content from your protocol under relevant journal-required headings. Then prewrite new material for results, limitations, discussion, and implications. Put off finalizing your conclusion, title, and abstract until the end. Plan to read your article again and again as you write and rewrite.

Some journals require use of *Reporting Guidelines | EQUATOR Network* (equator-network.org) [2]. Those *Guidelines* standardize reporting of randomized trials, observational studies, diagnostic/

prognostic studies, case reports, qualitative research, and more. Thus, even if you are not required to use EQUATOR, you might choose to do so in order to make sure you include key content. The benefit could be the difference between article acceptance or rejection.

12.3.4 Article Sections

Introduction includes a statement of the problem, its significance, and the purpose of your study. Follow this with a review of the literature that explains problem background, and then list your specific hypotheses/questions (H/Qs). The literature review includes what we know and don't know from existing research about the topic. What we don't know then leads to the H/Qs.

Procedures (Methods) should be detailed enough to facilitate study replication. The first sentence typically notes that "after IRB approval" you used a specified research design and instrument to collect data from a particular sample and setting. This is followed by your step-by-step actions in conducting the study: Intervention details, instrument description, subject recruitment and selection, and data collection and analysis. Identify analytic software. A box depicting the intervention or randomization process may help. Include the number of participant refusals or withdrawals if known, and note any mid-study changes. In qualitative studies, explain measures that you took to ensure dependability, credibility, confirmability, and transferability (earlier Box 5.4).

Results (Findings) sections differ for quantitative versus qualitative data studies. Qualitative researchers often integrate data analysis and interpretation in Results, while quantitative researchers document numerical results of statistical analyses under Results and the interpretation of those results in the Discussion section.

Tip. Look for examples in Results sections in other articles.

Start quantitative study Results with participant response rate—30% is often acceptable—and note whether or not any power analysis requirements were met. Follow this with statistical descriptions of sample demographics and of each outcome variable. In contrast, start qualitative Results with a thick, detailed description of informants that supports transferability. Both quantitative and qualitative reports may describe sample demographics statistically.

Next report qualitative or statistical test results for each H/Q and state whether or not hypotheses were supported or questions answered. Describe particular results either in the text or tables and graphs, not both. Stay within the number of figures, graphs, and tables allowed by the journal, and use required formatting.

Your statistical analysis printout shows the numerical values you need for reporting inferential results in text (Box 12.3). For descriptive results include measures of central tendency, distribution, and number of respondents used to calculate each (earlier Box 9.2). Find formatting for reporting more statistical tests online, or consult your statistician.

Box 12.3 Selected Statistical Reporting Format

Test	Typical format
Pearson's r; Spearman's rho (r)	$r(\text{df}) = $ [calculated r], $p = $ [calculated p][a]
t-test	$t(\text{df}) = $ [calculated t], $p = $ [calculated p]
ANOVA(F) within subjects[b]	F(df between groups, df within groups) = [calculated F], $p = $ [calculated p]
Chi-square (χ^2)	χ^2 (df, N=sample size) = [chi-square value], $p = $ [calculated p]
Mann-Whitney U (U)[c]	$U = $ [calculated U], $p = $ [calculated p]
Wilcoxon signed rank (Z)	$Z = $ [calculated Z], $p = $ [calculated p]
Kruskal-Wallis (H)	$H = $ [calculated H] (df), $p = $ [calculated p]

[a]df is degrees of freedom
[b]Because ANOVA tests for difference in ≥ 3 groups, conduct post hoc testing for statistically significant ANOVA results in order to identify which groups differ from each other. Common post hoc tests: Tukey, Newman-Keuls, Scheffee, Bonferroni, or Dunnett.
[c]z = [calculated z score] may be used instead of U = [calculated U]

For qualitative studies detail your analytic approach and outcome. For example, in a phenomenology study you might explain step-by-step application of Colaizzi's seven analytic steps and then report final results as the essence of informants' experience. Always support results with selected, illustrative informant comments, photographs, or other nonnumerical data.

Limitations include a brief summary of any quantitative study lack of generalizability, procedural issues, and poorly controlled extraneous variables. For qualitative studies limitations may include credibility, dependability, confirmability, and transferability issues.

> **Tip.** Transparency about limitations enables others to use your results wisely. Reality is complicated.

Discussion explains what your results mean without repeating them. In qualitative studies a separate Discussion section may be unnecessary or limited to a comparison with literature.

In quantitative studies, first make a case for the representativeness of your sample by comparing its demographics to those of the target population or eligible nonrespondents. This is important when interpreting a study's statistical, internal, and external validity. Then explain the results of each H/Q within the context of literature, your clinical knowledge, representativeness of the sample, strengths and weaknesses of procedures, and possible rival hypotheses. Reviewing earlier Box 6.2 may help. Include potential impact of any mid-study protocol changes on outcomes, and report tool reliability statistics using your own data. Again, transparency empowers readers to use findings well.

> **Alert!** Use tentative language, such as "findings suggest…" or "it may be that…." Avoid the word "prove" and its synonyms.

If results do *not* support your hypothesis, brainstorm possible reasons, such as limited control of extraneous variables. Point out results that may be clinically meaningful (clinically significant) to individuals, groups, or healthcare decisions. When findings are generalizable, rejecting hypotheses is as important as accepting them. Write in a way that preempts possible editorial bias against publishing studies that rejected hypotheses.

Tip from Thomas Edison. "I have not failed. I've just found 10,000 ways that won't work." [3]

Implications gives you an opportunity to describe the practical importance of findings for patients, families, clinicians, educators, researchers, or administrators and managers. Suggest ways that future researchers might remedy study limitations. When results are not generalizable exercise caution in making recommendations beyond proposing future research.

Conclusion often begins with a topic sentence summarizing the main study points and ends with a clear statement about next steps or your project's value. Look back at your first introductory paragraph for ideas, and never introduce new ideas in Conclusion. If you have a new idea, perhaps it belongs in Discussion.

Abstract word count and headings are specified by the journal. Refine the abstract you already wrote for IRB close-out or a conference. Remember that the abstract is a 30,000-foot-level view of your project, while the article is a ground-level, detailed perspective.

Keywords section is comprised entirely of three to five search terms that will lead others to your study. Paste your abstract into MeSH (Medical Subject Headings) on Demand (https://meshb.nlm.nih.gov/MeSHonDemand) to get a list of PubMed terms, or generate a few of your own.

Title should be written last. Remember to state it as a mini-abstract of your completed article including population, any intervention, key variable(s), and implied or explicit design.

Alert! Never use cause-and-effect words in your title unless you conducted an experiment.

12.3.5 Submit

Proof carefully. Never expect an editor to rewrite your article for you. They won't. Read only topic sentences to make sure content flows. Use your computer's read aloud function to listen to your article; revise as needed. Check accuracy of citations and references. Double check to make sure you have followed journal instructions in every detail, and then ask a mentor or peer to critique your work.

Tip. Submit your edited article only after you would be comfortable having it published as is.

Before uploading your article for peer review, do a final spelling and grammar check. Then allow time for the sometimes cumbersome process of submitting your article one piece at a time through journal software: The abstract, body, tables, and so on often are submitted as separate documents that the software converts into a complete article pdf file. Proof the pdf *before* clicking the final submit button.

Along with submission you will also complete conflict of interest forms, transfer copyright to the journal, and verify that your work is submitted only to them and not previously published. Be honest. These requests from credible journals are not a threat to your work, and if the journal rejects your article, copyright remains yours. If you have coauthors, ask them to designate you as corresponding author with the journal.

Coauthors must also complete conflict of interest forms and self-certify qualification for authorship before your article can be peer reviewed. Those qualifications include making significant contributions to the study idea or design, to data collection and analysis, and to drafting and approving the final article [4]. All authors are accountable for content. Use the optional Acknowledgment section to recognize those who facilitated your project but don't meet authorship criteria.

Journal instructions may indicate how soon you can expect a decision. Your article may be accepted, accepted with revisions, rejected with a request for rewriting, or rejected outright.

- If accepted as is, great! This is rare. Expect a few editorial changes.
- If accepted with revisions, respond to every concern and include a resubmission table that has verbatim peer-reviewers' comments in column 1 and your response to each in column 2.
- If not accepted and you are asked for a substantial rewrite, decide whether to rewrite or submit elsewhere. Whichever you choose, improve your article based on peer reviews.
- If rejected outright, use reviewer comments to correct deficiencies, and submit to a different journal after reformatting to the new

journal's author guidelines. Rewrite anything that reviewers didn't understand.

Tip. Do not take editorial decisions personally. Peer reviewers are critiquing your article not your character.

Editors reject articles for many reasons. Perhaps the journal just published another project like yours, or they receive a super-abundance of submissions, or your topic doesn't fit their audience. You may always appeal a decision, but that may or may not succeed. Enlist mentor help, and never be hostile.

Tip. List your manuscript on your resume as "in review" during peer review, then as "in press" after editorial acceptance, and then with a date after publication.

After article acceptance the editor will send you a final layout (*galley proofs*) right before publication. Review these minutely from title through references. Only correct mistakes, and return promptly. The time for general editing is long past. The journal may publish your article online before the final, corrected, print version. After printing, cite that version on your resume.

Tip. If your article is never accepted by any journal, consider online self-publication on a site like ResearchGate (https://www.researchgate.net/).

12.4 Conclusion

Celebrate! You did it! You have come full circle through the research process. You planned, conducted, and reported study results. Moreover, your work probably raised new questions, and I hope you can't wait to answer those in your next study.

Final Alert! "We can't know everything about anything until we know everything about everything." - Ron Highfield PhD (personal communication)

References

1. DOAJ. Directory of open access journals; 2024. https://doaj.org/. Accessed 9 March 2024.
2. The UK EQUATOR Centre, Centre for Statistics in Medicine, NDORMS, University of Oxford. Equator network: enhancing the quality and transparency of health research. https://www.equator-network.org/reporting-guidelines/. Accessed 9 March 2024.
3. Ratcliff S, editor. Oxford essential quotations. 14th ed; 2016. https://www.oxfordreference.com/. Accessed 24 May 2024.
4. International Committee of Medical Journal Editors. Defining the role of authors and contributors; 2024. https://www.icmje.org/recommendations/browse/roles-and-responsibilities/defining-the-role-of-authors-and-contributors.html. Accessed 14 March 2024.

Protocol Worksheet

13

Directions: This Worksheet is a guide for gathering protocol informa-tion. Institutional Review Board (IRB) protocol templates vary. Add spacing as needed. Complete this Worksheet in any order.

Title of Study (include population & main variable(s); avoid question format):

Principal Investigator (PI) (name, academic degrees, research train-ing completed (CE or school), prior research experience, & other research qualifications):

Other Investigators (same information as for PI):

School Project ☐ Yes ☐ No

- **Faculty advisor** (name, credentials, & school)

- **Research-site contact/mentor** (name, credentials, & position title)

- **University-Facility affiliation agreement** (needed before you start) ☐ Yes ☐ No

M. E. F. Highfield, *Doing Research*,
https://doi.org/10.1007/978-3-031-79044-7_13

Broad Purpose: (Write 1–2 sentences about the problem, issue, or question you observed and who is impacted.): "The purpose of this study is_____

_____

_____ "

PICOT.   [Note: I   &   C   are   variations   of   the   same independent variable.]

Element	Your project
P = patient population or problem	
I = intervention or involvement in a situation (or E = exposure to)	
C = comparison to the intervention if any	
O = outcome measured (dependent variable)	
T = timing of measurement	

Literature Search Terms derived from PICOT:

* Search terms:
* Search librarian-assisted? ☐ Yes ☐ No

Hypotheses or Research Questions (include PICOT elements)_____

_____

Quantitative Research Variable Summary (Not applicable to qualitative studies. You may need to complete later sections first. Add a row for each outcome variable):

Outcome (dependent) variable name	Dictionary or theoretical definition (conceptual definition)	Measurement tool (operational definition)	Type of data & analysis
EXAMPLE: Quality of nurses' work life in NICU	A balance between compassion satisfaction & compassion fatigue (Stamm, 2010)	ProQOL5 scale- 3 scores: compassion satisfaction, burnout, & secondary traumatic stress	Before & after comparison of ordinal data using unpaired t-testing

Extraneous Variables (If hypothesizing, list all factors that affect your outcome measure)

Extraneous variable	Method of control or description

Qualitative Research Variable Summary (Not applicable to quantitative research. You may need to complete later sections first):

Variable name	Design	Measurement	Type of data & analysis
EXAMPLE: ICU nursing subculture	Ethnography	• Interviews with investigator as instrument • Unit map & photographs • Observation of RN communications • Field notes	Qualitative. Analysis will compare findings to elements of Leininger's Transcultural Sunrise Enabler (model).

13.1 Current Literature

- **Current knowledge**
  - Combinations of search terms used (including MeSH)
  - Databases searched: ☐ CINAHL ☐ PubMed ☐ Another (specify)
  - Evidence-based clinical guidelines searched: ☐ Cochrane Collaboration
    ☐ CINAHL ☐ JBI ☐ Professional organizations (specify) _____ ☐ Another (specify) _____
  - Related facility policies/procedures (specify) _____
- **Significance of the issue**
  - Is the issue high impact? ☐ Yes ☐ No ☐ Maybe (*Explain or give reference*) _____
  - Is the issue widespread? ☐ Yes ☐ No ☐ Maybe (*Explain or give reference*) _____
  - Who will benefit from this study ☐ Patients ☐ Nurses ☐ Students/Educators ☐ Hospitals ☐ Community ☐ Other group or individuals (specify) _____
    [Note: List benefits under RISKS/BENEFITS section below.]

- **State of the art & science**
  - From your literature review, list key things we know:_____

  _____
  _____
  _____
  _____
  _____
  _____

- **Gap** (what we don't know): Given above summary, what knowledge gap does your project fill?_____

  _____

  - Do you need to adjust your PICOT to fill the gap? ☐ Yes ☐ No. If yes, adjusted PICOT=_____

  _____
  _____
  _____

- **Theory or framework** that defines and describes the relationships between variables in the proposed study. (See also above "Quantitative Variable Summary"section.)_____

  _____
  _____
  _____

13.2 Design

☐ Experimental/intervention study (RCT)
☐ Quasi-experimental/intervention study ☐ Another experiment (specify):_____
☐ Cohort ☐ Case control ☐ Correlational ☐ Descriptive ☐ Case study/ case series
☐ Mixed methods (circle those that apply): Triangulation, Embedded, Exploratory, Explanatory
☐ Historical
☐ Methodological
☐ Ideological (specify):_____

☐ Another (specify):_____

- Type of data to be collected: ☐ Quantitative ☐ Qualitative ☐ Both
- Timing: ☐ Prospective ☐ Retrospective ☐ Cross-sectional ☐ Longitudinal
- Data status: ☐ Existing data ☐ New data
- Research aim: ☐ Applied ☐ Basic

13.3   Risks, Resources, & Readiness (3R's)

Risks (List under Risk/Benefit later)

Resources Needed (LIST): ☐ Educator time ☐ Staff time ☐ Personnel ☐ Equipment ☐ Other Describe any in detail:

Readiness of Stakeholders: ☐ Faculty ☐ Clinical supervisor ☐ Research-site mentor ☐ Research-site committee ☐ Clinical educators ☐ Staff ☐ Interprofessional team members ☐ Research-site manager or staff (specify) _____ ☐ Other (specify)

_____

- Your plans to engage "unready" stakeholders? _____

_____

_____

_____

13.4   Procedures

Timeline: Anticipated dates and # of weeks for each phase after IRB approval (Modify Column 1 activities as needed).

Activities	Month/Year (# of weeks)
Sample recruitment	
Consent	
Pretest data collection	
Intervention	
Posttest data collection	
Analysis	
Dissemination	

Time Required of Each Subject During Participation

Activities (add rows prn)	**Hours: Minutes**
Example: Interview, intervention	60-90 minutes
Total time	

Intervention: ☐ Yes in hypothesis ☐ No

- Describe intervention:_____
- Describe comparison group treatments:_____
- Location of intervention?_____
- Any impact on those not in study? ☐ No ☐ Yes (descr
  ibe):_____
- Monetary cost of intervention to participants? ☐ No ☐ Yes (descr
  ibe):_____
- Participants compensated with money or services? ☐ No ☐ Yes
  (describe):_____
- Resources & contacts for subjects
  - If feel harmed_____
  - If study questions_____

Setting of data collection: ☐ Single site ☐ Multisite ☐ Laboratory
☐ School ☐ Healthcare institution ☐ Community ☐ Living space/
home ☐ Phone ☐ Other _____

- **Name of setting:**
- **Characteristics of named setting** (e.g., # of beds or patients
  treated per year, enrollment, etc.)

Sample
- Target population (e.g., age, sex, health status, etc.):_____
  _____

- Vulnerable population ☐ No ☐ Minors ☐ Cognitively impaired ☐ Prisoners ☐ Another (specify)_____
- Accessible population:_____
- Setting of sample recruitment _____
  _____

- Sample characteristics
  - ☐ Patients ☐ Providers ☐ Students ☐ Educators ☐ Documents (specify)_____ ☐ Another (specify)_____
  - Inclusion criteria_____
  - Exclusion criteria_____
- Sample size & rationale:☐ Power analysis ☐ Feasibility ☐ Qualitative study ☐ Other (specify)_____
  _____
  _____

- Sample selection procedures:
  - ☐ Non-probability/nonrandom (specify strategy):_____
  - ☐ Probability/random (specify strategy):_____
  - ☐ Randomization (random assignment to groups). Number of groups_____
  - ☐ Screening procedure for Ss eligibility? _____
  - Describe details of subject recruitment procedures, including when and how any recruitment material specified below will be used

- Recruitment materials (attach full final copy): ☐ None ☐ Posters/flyers/letters ☐ Email ☐ Social media ☐ In-person script ☐ Other (specify) _____

Instruments: (If Multiple Instruments, Add Rows)

- *Demographic* questionnaire if any (Attach copy) _____
  _____

- *Investigator-developed* instrument name (Attach copy) ._____
  _____
  - Validity documented ☐ Yes (specify)_____ ☐ No
  - Reliability documented ☐ Yes (specify)_____ ☐ No
  - Scoring described ☐ Yes (specify)_____ ☐ No
- *Copyrighted* instrument name (attach copy)_____
  _____

- Validity documented ☐ Yes (types)_____
  _____ ☐ No
- Reliability documented ☐ Yes (types)_____
  _____ ☐ No
- Scoring described ☐ Yes (specify)_____ ☐ No
- Documented permission to use ☐ Yes ☐ Not applicable (explain)
  _____
- Translation: ☐ Required ☐ Completed ☐ N/A (Describe)
  _____
- Reading level check: ☐ Required ☐ Completed ☐ N/A (Describe)_____
- Procedure for distribution & collection of instruments:
  _____

Raw Data Spreadsheet: [EXCEL or REDCap data entry recommended. Below is example spreadsheet]

Subject ID/MR#	Con-sent-ed	With-drew/ lost to f/u	Subject age in years	Subject ethnicity	Subject diagnosis	Survey question 1 rating	Survey question 2 rating	Etc.
Example 1	√		43	Hispanic	CML	3	5	etc.
2								

Data Analysis

- Total number of subjects (Ss)_____; Number of groups___; Number of subjects in each group_____
- Are subjects in each group ☐ same Ss ☐ different Ss
- If design is pretest/posttest, check one: ☐ Group pre/post averages compared (unpaired analysis); ☐ Individual pre/post scores compared (paired analysis)

Needed Analysis

- Quantitative, descriptive: ☐ Demographics ☐ Outcome variables
- Qualitative, descriptive: ☐ No ☐ Yes (specify major tradition and specific method in that tradition, e.g., "Phenomenology using Colaizzi's steps"):_____
  _____
- Inferential statistics: ☐ No ☐ Yes (specify):_____
- Preset significance level ☐ $p \leq 0.01$ ☐ $p \leq 0.05$ ☐ $p \leq 0.10$
- Analysis completed by ☐ Statistician ☐ Researcher (Note: if sent off-site describe data privacy protection): _____
  _____

Data Protection

- Collected data are ☐ Anonymous ☐ Confidential
- Briefly describe how Ss anonymity or confidentiality is maintained
  _____
  _____
  _____
- Who will access the data? ☐ Only researcher(s) ☐ Statistician
  ☐ Other (describe)_____
- Where will data be secured? ☐ Password protected computer
  ☐ Locked file/office ☐ REDCap or similar ☐ Other (describe)
  _____
- Data privacy protection if sent off-site for analysis or other (describe, e.g., encrypted email): _____
  _____
- How long will data be stored? Disposition/deletion of data by whom?
  _____
  _____
- Describe if data will be maintained for future research (describe & include in consent): _____
  _____

Consent

- Included sample:
  - Individuals with capacity over the age of 18? ☐ Yes ☐ No
  - Vulnerable population? ☐ Yes ☐ No
  - Describe special protections for any vulnerable population:_____

- Documentation of consent (attach full consent forms to IRB proposal) [Note: IRBs may provide consent forms requiring exact font size and information, or abbreviated form for minimal risk protocols]

  - Participant signature required ☐ Yes ☐ No
  - Consent or signature waived because: ☐ Signature is threat to privacy ☐ Cannot reasonably obtain signature ☐ Group or de-identified data ☐ Other_____
  - Consent script/form is in language of subjects ☐ Yes ☐ No ☐ N/A. Describe any translation:_____
  - Assent script/form is in language of subjects ☐ Yes ☐ No ☐ N/A. Describe any translation:_____
  - Legally authorized representative (LAR) signature required ☐ No ☐ Yes (explain)_____
  - Assent required ☐ No ☐ Yes (explain) _____

  _____

- Any deception used ☐ No ☐ Yes (Describe need for deception, minimal risk, and debriefing post data collection)_____
  _____

13.5 Risks/Benefits

Risks

- Risks to subjects & duration of each (check boxes that apply; add rows as needed)
  1. <u>Ss concern about being identified with responses:</u> ☐ Likely ☐ Unlikely **&** ☐ Mild ☐ Severe
  2. _____☐ Likely ☐ Unlikely **&** ☐ Mild ☐ Severe
  3. _____☐ Likely ☐ Unlikely **&** ☐ Mild ☐ Severe

- If any of above risks are not reversible, explain:_____
- How you will minimize each risk
    1. _____
    2. _____
    3. _____

Benefits

- Benefits to subjects (add rows as needed)
    1. _____☐ Likely ☐ Unlikely **&**
       ☐ Great or ☐ Minimal
    2. _____ ☐ Likely ☐ Unlikely **&**
       ☐ Great or ☐ Minimal
    3. _____☐ Likely ☐ Unlikely **&**
       ☐ Great or ☐ Minimal

- Benefits to others (e.g., family, future patients or nurses)
    1. _____☐ Likely ☐ Unlikely
    2. _____☐ Likely ☐ Unlikely
    3. _____☐ Likely ☐ Unlikely

- Benefits to organization/system
    1. _____☐ Likely ☐ Unlikely
    2. _____☐ Likely ☐ Unlikely
    3. _____☐ Likely ☐ Unlikely

- Do benefits **to subjects** outweigh risks **to subjects**? ☐ Yes ☐ No
  (You must be able to answer "yes.")

Appendices

Appendix A

Literature Search Guidelines

1st. **Formulate a list of key words from your PICOT**. Do *not* use general terms like "inpatient" or "illness." If you do, you'll get thousands of useless articles. Keep terms tightly focused on a narrow PICOT population, setting, intervention, and outcome. For example, "animal assisted therapy," "motivation," and/or "spinal cord injury."

   Access a healthcare library online or in person. If you are a student or staff, you'll have access to many databases to which the library subscribes. You can search without student or staff privileges, but you won't be able to retrieve as much information as quickly, and you may need to buy articles. You can retrieve free "open access" articles, but verify their credibility by checking the Directory of Open Access Journals (DOAJ).

2nd. Start by looking for the strongest types of research evidence: Systematic reviews, meta-analyses, and evidence-based guidelines (Fig. 5.1). These expert-syntheses of evidence are *secondary, filtered research* or *pre-appraised research*.

   Find relevant evidence-based practice guidelines in:

   - A pull down menu at the top of the database page;
   - Professional organization websites; and
   - Health-related government websites (.gov).

© The Author(s), under exclusive license to Springer Nature Switzerland AG 2025 111
M. E. F. Highfield, *Doing Research*,
https://doi.org/10.1007/978-3-031-79044-7

Search PubMed, the Joanna Briggs Institute (JBI), the Cochrane Collaboration, and the Cumulative Index of Nursing & Allied Health Literature (CINAHL) using your search terms and "systematic review" OR "meta-analysis," OR "evidence based guidelines." Include "OR" between terms to tell the database that any one of the linked terms is okay.

If you do find an applicable systematic review, meta-analysis, or EBP guideline, check the date of publication. Obtain a copy of it and of individual research reports published after that date.

Use optional Boolean operators to limit or expand your search, including:

- Quotation marks that prompt the database to find articles with the phrase, not the individual words (e.g., "animal assisted therapy").
- An asterisk after a partial term that prompts the database to retrieve any form of your truncated word; for example nurs* will retrieve articles with nurse, nursing, nurses, and so on.
- Using the word AND between terms tells the database that you want only publications that have all the linked terms; using it limits your search results. Using OR tells a database that you want articles with any of the terms; using it expands search results.
- Using the word NOT tells the database any terms that you want to exclude and can be used to narrow a search by excluding irrelevant material.

Tip. Numerous tutorials for searching major database PubMed are online (https://www.youtube.com/playlist?list=PL7dF9e2q SW0YkmxDTsUG6p4hJjYOPT0Uj)

3rd. Next use your key terms and any Boolean operators to search credible, comprehensive databases, like CINAHL and PubMed for *primary, unfiltered reports*. Primary, unfiltered studies are single studies written by their original authors. Limit your search to the past three to five years.

Use Boolean operators AND, OR, and NOT as needed. Narrow a search by adding more terms or searching fewer years, and expand it by dropping terms, trying synonyms, expanding years, or reviewing reference lists in retrieved articles. Keep track of the combinations you use.

If you find only old studies, search for new publications that cite those.

The FAQ page on the free PubMed database (https://pubmed.ncbi.nlm.nih.gov/help/) describes many best search practices, such as using Boolean operators (e.g., AND, *, NOT, OR) and how to save, expand, share, or restrict a search. PubMed also has a free tutorial on its Medical Subject Headings (MeSH) that are terms used to index articles.

CINAHL has a "Help" link and an "Advanced" search link beneath the search boxes that allows you to limit your search as needed, for example by years, peer-reviewed, and language. You can limit type of publication to systematic reviews, meta-analysis, or evidence based guidelines.

Finally, a quick internet search may yield numerous free, full-text articles, websites, and videos of varying scientific quality. Search engine Google Scholar and ResearchGate may contain both published reports and *grey literature.* Grey literature is not peer-reviewed and includes government or association reports, white papers, and working documents. Much grey literature is expert opinion or background—useful, but weak evidence. ResearchGate (researchgate.net) also contributes a network of researchers interested in your topic.

Alert! Do not rely only on *search engines* like Bing or Google Scholar. They are limited, hit-and-miss sites that are not linked to professional databases. They both leave much undiscovered and include predatory journals.

4th. Save relevant articles or references or email them to yourself. Download those with full text to your personal device, and request the others via interlibrary loan. Links for these functions are within databases or library pages.

Alert! Never save your username and password on any public computer and be sure to log out.

Appendix B

Editable Script for Consent Information (See IRB Requirements for Full Information)

Page 1 of [Total # of Consent Pages]

This research study is conducted by [investigator name and affiliation]. The purpose of the study is to [broad purpose/aim/questions].

I am asking you for voluntary [completion of questionnaire/other participation]. I am contacting you as a potential research study participant because you are [eligibility criteria], and I located your name/ contact information through [process/document/person].

If you agree to participate in this project, you will be asked to [activity including who, what, when, where, how, how long]. This will take [total time and number of interactions with the researcher during and after the study]. You may choose to continue or stop our contact at any time for any reason either verbally or in writing.

The benefits of participating in this project include [list benefits]. You may benefit from knowing that you helped to improve care for others or find the process personally empowering, transformative, and sometimes healing. [Note: This is an example. Write only what applies.]

Potential risks of participating in the project include [list risks]. To minimize these risks, [list actions taken to minimize each risk]. [For interviews add "You may also elect to use a pseudonym instead of your real name," and be sure to include any possible risks of others still being able to identify them.]

You will neither pay nor be paid to participate. When the study is completed you will also be able to request a project report by contacting [investigator/other].

If you are concerned about the research, you may direct questions to [IRB contact information]. If you have specific questions about the study you may contact [investigator contact information/other study personnel].

You should understand that your consent to participate in this study is completely voluntary. You may decline to participate or withdraw from the study at any time without penalty or explanation. Likewise the investigator may cancel this study at any time.

If you withdraw from this study, [list harms] may occur. To minimize that harm [list investigator actions for each harm].

I have read the above, had my questions answered and understand the conditions outlined for participation in the described study. I have also received a copy of this form.

[Participant signature and date, and Investigator signature and date]

Glossary

Accessible population A readily available subset of the target population.

Assent The agreement to participate in a study by persons who cannot legally grant consent, such as children or cognitively impaired adults.

Assumptions Propositions assumed to be true as a basis for a study. They are not tested in the study.

Bias, systematic Consistent bias in sampling or data collection that creates distorted results, such as a non-calibrated instrument that overestimates values.

Bias, random Bias in a study related to shifting variations in the sample, environment, researcher, or an unreliable measurement instrument.

Bivariate analysis Statistical analysis of the relationship between two variables.

Blinding Procedures to prevent researchers from identifying who is receiving the intervention.

Bracketing When qualitative researchers identify and set aside their own biases that may affect data collection, analysis, and reporting.

Case controlled study Participants with and those without a disease or condition are compared in terms of their exposure to a presumed cause.

Cleaning data (see Data cleaning)

Clinical significance (or clinical importance or clinical meaningfulness) The observable, practical impact of an intervention on clinical care of some individuals, groups, or healthcare decisions, whether or not the effect of the intervention was statistically significant.

© The Author(s), under exclusive license to Springer Nature Switzerland AG 2025
M. E. F. Highfield, *Doing Research*,
https://doi.org/10.1007/978-3-031-79044-7

Cohort study Participants with variable amounts of exposure to a presumed cause are followed to identify emerging health issues or retrospectively to determine the amount of exposure related to outcomes.

Conceptual definition A dictionary-type definition of a variable.

Concurrent validity A methodological measure of tool accuracy in which scores on different instruments measuring the same construct at the same time are expected to be similar.

Consent (see Informed consent and Process consent)

Constant comparison When qualitative data are analyzed as they are collected.

Construct validity A measure of how accurately a tool measures what it is supposed to measure.

Content analysis Examining any text, interviews, or other documents to identify emerging or recurrent concepts and sometimes the relationship between concepts.

Content validity A measure of how comprehensively tool items represent a given concept/construct. Determined by expert panel or calculation of content validity index (CVI).

Continuous data Data measured in whole and fractional numbers on a continuum.

Convenience sampling Non-random, non-probability selection of subjects who are thus unlikely to represent a larger target population.

Correlational study Research examining a statistical association between two or more variables.

Co-variate (co-variable) A variable not of direct interest but that can affect the dependent variables.

Criterion-related validity A measure of how well a new tool's measurement correlates with a known standard measurement. May be predictive or concurrent.

Cross-sectional study Study with data collection at a single time point or points close together.

Data (sing. datum) A collection of multiple, separate word or numerical measurements of a given variable.

• **Nominal data:** Data that can be counted only in categories without any mathematical value.

• **Ordinal data:** Data that can be placed in a meaningful order, but without equal intervals between values.

- **Interval data:** Data that can be placed in meaningful order with equal intervals between values, but no absolute zero.
- **Ratio data:** Data that can be placed in a meaningful order with equal intervals between values and an absolute zero.

Data cleaning   Preparing quantitative data for analysis by dealing with inconsistent labels, outliers, and missing data.

Data integrity   Accuracy and completeness of data without corruption.

Data saturation   When respondents surface no new ideas within an interview or in an ongoing series of interviews. Part of grounded theory concurrent data collection and analysis.

Data security   Measures to protect data from access by unauthorized persons.

Debriefing   The reversal of any investigator deception; when the investigator gives accurate and full information to subjects after data collection and reaffirms consent.

Deception   During consent when the investigator provides only partial information or misleading information about a study in order to prevent subjects from conforming responses to what they think the researchers want to know.

Deductive reasoning   Drawing conclusions about specific situations from general theory.

Dependent variable   The outcome that is measured; also called effect or outcome variable.

Descriptive study   Qualitative or quantitative study of the natural characteristics or occurrence of one or more variables without researcher intervention.

Digital commons   A worldwide online space where facility-specific scholarly materials are posted.

Discrete data   Data measured as categories and whole numbers.

Disproportionate sampling   Over-sampling of smaller segments of a population in order to secure adequate representation in all groups. Contrast with proportionate sampling.

Effect size   Statistical calculation of the magnitude of the effect of one variable on another or the strength of a relationship between variables.

Emic observation   Participating in an event or group and observing them as an insider.

Etic observation   Observing as an outsider to events or groups.

Evidence-based practice (EBP)   Best clinical practice grounded in best scientific evidence, clinical judgment, and patient/family preferences and values.

Evidence-informed quality improvement (EBQI)   When scientific evidence is the basis for quality improvement activity.

Extraneous variables   Factors outside of study hypotheses or questions that may affect study outcomes if they are not controlled.

Extreme case sampling   In qualitative research, sampling of those who represent outermost ends of the phenomenon being studied.

Face validity   Expert judgment that a data collection tool measures what it purports to measure.

Factor analysis   In methodological studies, the statistical categorizing of like items into groups called factors. Used to support construct validity of an instrument.

Generalizability   The extent to which findings of a study can reasonably be applied to the target population or a similar sample and setting.

Grey literature   Credible documents published outside peer-reviewed sources, such as white papers from professional organizations or government.

Hawthorne effect   When subjects alter their behavior simply because they are being studied.

History bias   Distortion in research results created by events immediately before or concurrent with a study.

Homogenous sample   Sampling of persons who are the same in regard to key variables. In qualitative research, contrast with maximum variation.

Human Subjects Review Board   (see Institutional review board)

Hypothesis   An evidence-based prediction about the relationship between two or more variables.

Informant   Typically meaning a subject in a qualitative study; implies exercise of subject agency.

Independent variable   The researcher-manipulated intervention; also called the causative variable.

Inductive reasoning   Building theory by developing generalizations from specific observations.

Informed consent   Voluntary agreement to participate in a study based on comprehension of researcher-provided, complete information.

Institutional review board An institutionally-convened group of professionals and patient advocates charged with protecting human research subjects by approving only research protocols that meet legal and regulatory requirements as well as institutional policies.

Intense sampling Qualitative sampling of those who most powerfully experienced the phenomenon.

Legally authorized representative Entity or person who can consent to a study on behalf of another.

Longitudinal study A study with multiple data collection points from the same population over a long period of time, even years to decades.

Maximum variation sampling Qualitative sampling of those experiencing every possible variation of the phenomenon.

Mediating variable A variable between cause and effect variables that has a direct causal effect on the outcome variable.

Member checks Post-analysis validation of findings with qualitative study informants.

Minimal risk study Research in which risk is the same as in activities of daily life or in routine, individual testing.

Mixed methods study Collection and integrated analysis of quantitative and qualitative data.

Moderating variable A variable between cause and effect variables that is not part of the cause, but instead shifts the strength or direction of changes in the outcome.

Multi-variate analysis Statistical analysis of the relationships between three or more variables.

Non-probability sampling Non-random subject selection in which some members of a population are more likely to be chosen as study participants.

Null (statistical) hypothesis An assumption of inferential statistics that there is no difference between control and experimental group outcomes.

Operational definition A data collection tool that measures the conceptual definition of a variable.

Outlier data Measurements of a variable that are extremely high or low in comparison to measurements from most participants.

Panel study In a longitudinal study when the same persons are subjects at every data collection point.

Participant observation   In observational, often qualitative studies when the data collector functions as a member of the group under observation in order to get an insider (emic) perspective.

Phenomenon (pl. phenomena)   An event or experience often represented in a single word or phrase (e.g., insomnia or losing a job). An abstraction that can be translated into measurable characteristics.

Phenomenology   Qualitative study that aims to document the "lived experience" of those who have experienced a phenomenon and can articulate that experience.

Pilot study   Small-scale study that aims to test research procedures before using them in a larger, full-scale study.

Population   (see Target population or Accessible population)

Power analysis   A statistical calculation of the needed sample size for an experimental study.

Presentism   Interpreting historical data within the researcher's present context rather than in the data's historical context.

Primary source   An original article; or a person with direct, first-hand knowledge of something; or a document produced at the time of a historical situation being studied.

Principal investigator (PI)   The lead researcher on a study. Co-principal investigators may jointly lead a study.

Probability sampling   Random subject selection so that any member of the population is equally likely to be chosen as a participant.

Process consent   A qualitative researcher's discretionary reaffirmation of informant consent during an interview in order to avoid the informant's unplanned sharing of illegal or especially senitive information.

Prolonged engagement   Researchers' engagement with subjects over an extended period of time.

Proportionate sampling   Sampling from different segments of the population in the same proportions that those segments naturally occur within the population.

Proposition   A statement about one concept/variable or about the relationship between two or more concepts/variables

Purposive (or judgment) sampling   A researcher's handpicked, nonrandom selection of those who experienced and can articulate their experiences with the phenomenon of interest.

Quantitative research A study in which the research question or hypothesis is answered with numerical data.

Qualitative research A study in which the research question is answered with non-numerical data.

Quasi-experiment Researchers test an intervention without randomization and/or a control group. An example is single group, pretest/posttest.

Random sampling (see Probability sampling)

Randomization Randomly assigning members of a sample to control or experimental group(s).

Randomized controlled trial (RCT) A true experiment. Researchers randomly assign participants to control or experimental groups and test an intervention.

Raw data Data prior to analysis.

REDCap Research Electronic Data Capture software for secure online data collection and analysis.

Reflexivity Researcher reflection on how one's own biases and context may affect a study and interpretation of findings.

Researcher-as-instrument When the data collector becomes part of qualitative data collection, such as during an interview when the researcher modifies questions or follows up on participant leads.

Response set bias Respondents propensity to provide data in the same general direction. Four main types are:

• **Acquiescence bias:** Tendency to agree no matter what the question.

• **Extreme bias:** Regularly giving "always" and "never" answers.

• **Neutrality bias:** Consistently giving a middle, "maybe," non-committal answer.

• **Social desirability bias:** Answering to portray oneself in the best light possible.

Rigor The strength of a research study based on its adherence to sound scientific principles and control of extraneous variables and biases.

Rival hypothesis A competing explanation for study results in which an extraneous variable not the researcher-controlled intervention created study outcomes.

Sampling (see Probability sampling and non-probability sampling)

Sampling frame   List of all people or things from which a sample will be drawn.

Secondary source   A person or resource with second-hand, indirect knowledge of something.

Selection bias   When a selected or retained sample is distorted toward certain characteristics and so does not represent the target population. Bias may be random or systematic.

Skewed curve   When subject data cluster together on either extreme end of possible scores rather than forming a normal bell-shaped curve.

Strata (sing. stratum)   Divisions in a population based on age, ethnicity, or another characteristic.

Target population   The broad group to whom you want to generalize the results from your sample.

Theory-based sampling   In qualitative research, a sampling method that seeks to represent all concepts within a theory about the phenomenon being studied.

Thick description   In qualitative research a detailed, in-depth description of informants.

Transferability   In qualitative research a judgment about how accurately results can be applied to others.

Trend study   At each data collection point in a longitudinal study, researchers draw a different sample from the larger population they are following.

Triangulation   Triangulation is using more than one data source to verify accuracy of data or more than one researcher to verify accuracy of analysis.

Typical case sampling   In qualitative research a sampling strategy of selecting those most archetypal of those experiencing the phenomenon of interest.

Research design   The overall plan for answering the research question or hypothesis.

Research Question   Asked when not enough evidence exists to hypothesize; a question about some variable(s) of interest.

Univariate analysis   Statistical analysis of one variable.

Variable   A measurable concept that can vary and so holds different values.

Bibliography

1. Bevans R. Choosing the right statistical test. Types & Examples; 2020/2023. https://www.scribbr.com/statistics/statistical-tests/. Accessed 3 October 2024.
2. Creswell J. John Creswell YouTube Channel; n.d. https://www.youtube.com/@johncreswell6094/featured. Accessed 9 March 2024.
3. Davies B, Logan J. Reading research: a user-friendly guide for health professionals. 7th ed. Toronto: Elsevier; 2021.
4. Excelsior University. Excelsior Online Writing Lab (OWL); 2023. https://owl.excelsior.edu/writing-process/prewriting-strategies. Accessed 27 March 2024.
5. Khan Academy. Statistics & probability; 2024. https://www.khanacademy.org/math/statistics-probability. Accessed 3 October 2024.
6. Kansas University Medical Center. Determination of quality improvement versus research; 2019. https://www.kumc.edu/documents/research-administration/irb/Quality-Improvement-vs-Research.pdf. Accessed 3 October 2024.
7. Leslie Becker Channel. Prewriting strategies. In YouTube; 2017. https://www.youtube.com/watch?v=OQJSrQT9loI. Accessed 9 March 2024.
8. Owens JK, Chinn P. Reference letters and the specter of publications in predatory journals. Nurse Author & Editor. 2018;28:2.
9. National Institutes of Health. How to write a Data Safety and Monitoring Plan (DSMP); 2024. https://www.niams.nih.gov/grants-funding/conducting-clinical-trials/clinical-trial-policies-guidelines-and-templates/data-and. Accepted 7 October 2024.
10. Rees C. Rapid research methods for nurses, midwives and health professionals. Hoboken, NJ: Blackwell; 2016.
11. Salkind NJ, Frey BB. Statistics for people who (think they) hate statistics. 7th ed. Thousand Oaks, CA: Sage; 2019.
12. Trochim WMK. Conjointly: research methods knowledge base; 2024. https://conjointly.com/kb/. Accessed 9 March 2024.
13. Trochim WMK, Donnelly JP. The research methods knowledge base. 3rd ed. Atomic Dog, Cengage Learning: Mason, OH; 2008.

14. UNESCO International Institution for Higher Education in Latin American and the Caribbean. ChatGPT and artificial intelligence in higher education: quick start guide; 2023. https://www.iesalc.unesco.org/wp-content/uploads/2023/04/ChatGPT-and-Artificial-Intelligence-in-higher-education-Quick-Start-guide_EN_FINAL.pdf?fbclid=IwAR1co3FyuvdJvECw80Thq7dtuzNxQk3ET2w9iFepo_x6TUI1_hsIvr1pTfk. Accessed 9 March 2024.

15. US Food & Drug Administration. Science & research; 2023. https://www.fda.gov/science-research. Accessed 4 October 2024.

Index